The Dorian Gray Diet

Inma Hannah

Note to the reader

This book is primarily aimed at adults with no particular health problems. The author urges that anyone with a medical condition which includes pregnancy, to consult their medical practitioner before using this book. The opinions in this book are entirely the authors own. References to studies are not given although are available, due to this not being an academic work, as it is written in the context of a self help book. Whilst every care has been taken to ensure the accuracy of the content, the author and the publishers cannot accept legal responsibility for any problems arising from following the methods set out in this publication.

Forward

The title of this book is meant to be tongue in cheek although it exemplifies the content and the aims of this book, that is to appear younger than your age would say you are. This has also been a passing comment to us on occasions, so an apt title in all respects.

The content is a thoroughly straight forward 'how to' reduce, eliminate and contain the elements of ageing through diet and most importantly, correct food preparation. We have practiced this method from a crude beginning to the refined one you will see in the following pages. You may be skeptical or you may have followed other diet programs and not obtained the results you had hoped. This program, by it's nature – and you will realise soon enough – cannot and will not fail you.

This may be the most powerful diet and food preparation book you may ever see because of it's properties to rejuvenate. The linking in this book of the correct food **and** method of preparation is entirely new.

What is different about this way of living than any other diet publication that is invariably out there? Several reasons, which are explained in detail in the chapters that follow but suffice to say for each reason given, an explanation, a meal and preparation suggestion is given.

You will literally start to get the benefits written about, as soon as you have eaten the example meal that accompanies every section. A sort of eat as you learn reinforcement of the principles, certainly an enjoyable way to learn if there ever was one.

Another consideration and guiding principle is that this is all done with 'normal' food, no exclusive, expensive or hard to get items; everything is available via a good supermarket and an optional handful of items from a health food store, and that's your shopping done – and probably a lot more economically than what you are purchasing now.

A 'get you started' list of tasty recipes are in the appendix of which some them will be new to you and also, some old classic ones too, that are perfect for our purpose.

This book is written in simple to understand english. It is our belief that the content should be understood so that you can act on it with the confidence of **why** you are changing your food and the **way** you consume that food.

As a final note, the author who has followed this program for many years, is 'middle aged' and yet has no cellulitis, grey hair or wrinkles anywhere; is easily mistaken for someone in their early thirties and has a perfect figure. How would I know? - I am her husband of 18 years. What you waiting for? - read on!

Dominic Hannah

Mieres, Asturias

Table of Contents

Table of Contents

Introduction

These days, most of us want to be like Dorian Gray. It sounds like magic ! Keeping ourselves young while our portrait is growing old in the attic !

Feeling good with ourselves first thing in the morning when we go to the mirror, hearing the phrase "you haven't changed at all" when we meet someone we haven't seen for many years, going for a job interview or for a job promotion full of confidence knowing that we look much younger that they expect us to be, being called young lady or young man by someone who is only three or four years older than us, and so on. It is all these little things and many others that grow the confidence in us and give us the power to get what we want.

It is this *"Feel good"* factor that makes most of us to want the magic of making and keeping ourselves young. So badly we want it, that more and more people every year decide to undergo some kind of treatment (though we all know that these treatments never last).

But believe me, there is no magic after all ! You can be like Dorian Gray ! And you certainly don't have to sell your soul to the devil in order to achieve this !

You are ageing faster than you are supposed to and you can look 10 or in some situations, 20 years younger than you do at this moment. The correct diet will prevent your early ageing and it will repair the skin tissues already damaged.

Like most of you, I did not want to age either. It was my desire to stay young and my skepticism and fear of any treatment that involves needles and/or surgery that drew me into this research.

I did not like the bags I was getting under my eyes, (I learned later that although I was sleeping 8 hours, my sleep was not deep enough and it was to do with my wrong diet) neither I did I like the wrinkles I was getting around my eyes.

I wanted to get rid of all these unwanted things around my eyes, but I wanted the problem solved in a lasting way. So I was not very keen on aesthetic treatment that hide the problems on a temporary basis and don't regenerate or repair the skin, neither preventing further ageing.

It was all these discontents with myself and the fact that I wanted a genuine and a lasting solution, that convinced me to search for the reasons of ageing and it's process. From this, I started to take all the facts and apply them to my diet. Now, I am 42 and I have no wrinkles, no bags under my eyes, and no grey hair.

It is people's assumption that wrinkles and loose skin among many other symptoms, are unavoidable and just part of the natural process of ageing once you reach 30 plus, that convince them to either give up on themselves or to undergo to some kind of treatment, or nasty and helpless procedure, as to what they believe is the only and final resort.

Except this is not the case. From teenagers to 60 plus, every one is ageing before time and it has got nothing to do with your age; but with the number of years that you have been taking the wrong actions. Although you may try to avoid most of the free radicals (exposure to the sun, binge drinking, environmental stress, smoking, lack of sleep and so on) you are still constantly exposing yourself to major ones. These major ones are the free radicals you encounter in your daily food and drink intakes.

I decided to call these *major* free radicals, because you are constantly exposed to them more than you are exposed to any others (minimum 3 to 4 times a day) due to our own biological requirement. Even those who try, and believe they eat a healthy diet, do not realise they are still exposing themselves to these major free radicals.

This then, is where you need to focus, on the part that you do wrong with your daily intake of food and drink.

Although for some of you it could be your entire food and diet that needs to be changed, for many, it could just be the way you prepare it and/or combine it that makes it become a free radical meal.

Most important of all is, with the help of this book, you can say goodbye to all of the unwanted imperfections from your face and body. The ageing process you are going through is not the natural ageing process. You are ageing before time, and all the symptoms of ageing acceleration can be reversible through the correct diet.

Your body system is programmed to **self-repair** (limiting the damage your cells receive during your life time) and this function is carried out naturally by your own cells. It is your wrong eating habits and diet, that are the major factor why your cells stop conducting their own functions, causing consequently, the ageing acceleration process.

Our Cells

This is more basic that what you probably think. And many of you may be still remembering the subject from school, but never took much notice of it at the time.

At a microscopic level our body system is no more than an enormous number of cells. When we look ourselves in the mirror, what we see is the result of billions of cells which comprise of around 200 different types.

Our skin is made of skin cells, our livers are made of liver cells etc, as with every part of the body. The body is governed by specific types of cells.

In other words, the condition of your skin depends on the condition of your skin cells, as your skin condition, is nothing more but the reflection of your cells.

As we have already mentioned, our cells are programmed to self-repair themselves naturally (as their main function). So you will be asking yourself: Why am I ageing quickly?

and why are my cells not doing the self-repair job they are programmed to do so in the first place?.

We observe daily that once we have reached 30 or 35 years of age, the majority of people, men and women, experience a loss of hair thickness, grey hair, wrinkles on the face and stomach, bags under the eyes, loose skin in the face and body, flabby arms, cellulite etc. And some people's bodies, even if slim, are still feeling heavy and asleep!

The loose skin on your face and body is due to poor muscle tone. Even if you try to maintain yourself slim, your skin tends to end flaccid and not firm. Swollen eyelids and bags under your eyes are symptoms of a malfunction of your liver and/or kidney. And the pale and/or yellow skin complexion and chronic tiredness that you experience every day; are the symptoms of an overloaded pancreas.

All this evidence clearly indicates that your cells have stopped functioning properly. They are not executing any longer their main and natural function of self-repair, and by not being able to achieve this, all the damage taking place among them, has been accumulated in the tissues, making it visual in your skin, all the symptoms of the early degeneration process you are going through (or accelerating ageing in your skin).

But your cells can only fail to execute their main function, when an alteration and deterioration has occurred between them. This alteration and deterioration of your cells occurs when certain obstacles stand in the way, and these obstacles are the ones we call free radicals.

Biologically, our body is programmed to take care of these obstacles and your food intake is the combustible required by the body in order to battle and minimise free radicals. The problem is that you are replacing the combustible used by the body (food full of nutrients and substances) to combat free radicals with yet more free radicals (those encountered in your wrong daily food and drink intake).

In short, cells need food full of nutrients and substances in order to combat free radicals, but all you are doing by ingesting the wrong food, is confronting your body with more free radicals. This is the reason why you are ageing before time.

So this is what this program is all about.

This is not a weight loss diet program (though you will loose unwanted fat by eating the right foods) but a program to allow your cells to carry out their own functions without any obstacles standing on the way.

Essentials nutrients and substances will do wonders on your face and body. It will limit the damage that your cells will receive during a life time, and it will heal those that have already been damaged; and so you will be regaining a young a healthy skin once again

This program has been arranged in just 200 hundred pages written in simple English for everyone to understand in order to facilitate the facts of why you are ageing before time, how to prevent it and how to regenerate the damage already done.

On the first part of the book you will learn how to stop the ageing acceleration process that you are experiencing in your face and body and how to reverse the damage already done to your skin. On the second part you will get to know the reasons why you are ageing faster than you are supposed to and in the third and final part, we encounter all the instructions and adjustments to follow in order to achieve a full skin rejuvenation.

Note well, there is no magic but common sense! We can all be like Dorian Gray.

PART 1

How To Stop Ageing Acceleration

Cells require basic nutrients and essential substances in order to carry out their own functions without any obstacles standing in the way. Thus, eating foods enriched with vitamins, minerals, antioxidants, good fats and most of all with enzymes.

All of these nutrients are indispensable to your cells. This is because they participate in one way or another in every single reaction that takes place within the billions or trillions of cells in the body. They strengthen the immune system, they stop cell destruction caused by free radicals, they heal and promote new cell growth.

Remember that the skin is nothing more but the reflection of cells and as long as your cells receive all the substances they require, they will be able to perform their own functions. Not only you will be able to restore your skin and make it firmer by providing the right substances to your cells, but you will also have more energy and feel ill less frequently.

So, lets start to do things properly! which I would guess, is completely the opposite to what you have being doing until now. It is only by providing your cells with the right nutrients and avoid eating the wrong food that you will be able to prevent the accelerating ageing process you are going through at this moment, and restore the damage already caused to your skin.

Chapter1   Enzymes

Among all the nutrients and substances, I decided to begin with enzymes. This is because enzymes are indispensable for the absorption and digestion of all nutrients and minerals from your food, and it is the lack of enzymes in your daily food intake that is one of the main reasons why you are ageing faster than you are supposed to.

During the digestion process, enzymes tear apart in small particles all the food ingested in order to be absorbed easily by the body and transported to the bloodstream. These particles are the components that our body utilise as a combustible for the growth and reproduction of cells and also to repair the cells already damaged.

All enzymes are proteins and they participate in every function of the body. No only they are essential for the body's metabolism, but they also cleanse the body, breaking down allergens and environmental products that can potentially be harmful - free radicals - and cause cell destruction.

Enzymes are vital for the skin and bone structure, immune protection, muscles contraction and so on. Eighty percent of our DNA code relates to enzymes and as long as our cells obtain all the enzymes they require, they will be able to perform correctly and so growth and self-repair function will be carried out. Meaning, you will be able to replace a saggy skin with a firm one, avoid diseases and illnesses, and increase your vitality and longevity.

In other words, enzymes are the secret of youthfulness, vitality and longevity as they make possible the absorption and transportation of all nutrients and substances that cells require to carry out their functions.

How to Obtain our Enzymes

Proteins or enzymes (similar thing) are made of a long chain of amino acids. Among all the amino acids, 8 of them are indispensable (they are called essentials) and they must be supplied from food as they can not be made by the body.

These eight essential amino acids are:

> Valine, Threonine, Phenylalanine
> Isoulecine, Leucine, Tryptophan
> Methionine, Lysine

The others are not indispensable and so they are called non essentials, as the body has the ability to synthesize them from other amino acids through the correct diet.

All food contains some proteins (enzymes), each of them with their own amino acids composition. The proportion of each of the 8 essential amino acids in foods may differ from the proportions needed by the body to make proteins. And it is only the right combination and preparation of food that will make proteins to work efficiently and able to be used for growth and self repair.

Animal proteins contain all the essential amino acids in the proportion required by the body. So you would probably think that consuming food such as meat, cheese and milk, it would supply you with the proportion of protein required. Some people even tend to exceed four or five times the recommended daily amount of protein by having too much consumption of meat and dairy (see page 35 for recommended daily amount of protein intake) in the hope of gaining firmer skin.

But it is much more subtle than that. There are two major factors that prevent these kinds of proteins from working efficiently and they are the main reason why you are ageing before time.

One is the high temperature (proteins are very delicate substances and temperatures above 105 degrees C. (100 degrees C is boiling water) destroy proteins and nutrients from food) at which these foods are exposed during the cooking process. The other, is the type of protein combination. Protein can only work efficiently if energy needs are also met.

When energy needs are not met, proteins will have to be used for energy instead of tissue growth and repair. Normally the body uses a combination of protein and carbohydrate (from plants) or protein and natural sugars (derived from fruit) as a source of energy.

But the energy source that meat and dairy products contain consist of a combination of protein and saturated fat (bad fat). With the largest part of meat and dairy consisting of protein, the body will have to use protein as a source of energy instead of using it for tissue growth and repair.

So not only has the protein content of meat and dairy products been destroyed throughout the cooking process and/or pasteurisation, but this conversion of protein into energy is more difficult and takes much more energy, (6 to 8 hours to digest) than the conversion of carbohydrate and/or natural sugars into energy; which only takes 30 minutes to digest.

As a result of both, your pancreas ends up being overloaded and exhausted after so much work. Energy from protein and other resources is spent in digesting the food, instead of being used as the supply required by your cells in order to conduct their own functions such as growth, repair, increasing your immune system and combating cell destruction and illnesses.

Therefore, instead of providing the nutrients that your cells require, you are making your body exhausted by over expending energy and resources during the process of digestion.

Thus, you speed up your ageing process by deteriorating your body much faster than it is supposed to. And it is no only your skin that is suffering. As time goes by, after a repetitive consumption of food consisting of bad fats and no energy, your pancreas begins to expand and inflame and your organs began to loose balance. Various investigations have demonstrated that this is the cause of many degenerative diseases.

Low levels of energy in protein food intake have been associated with deficiencies of hormonal tissues (including that of the thyroid hormone) ,susceptibility to a number of viruses, infections and allergies, constant chronic fatigue and osteoporosis.

In short, meat and dairy products lack enzymes and contain saturated fats (bad fats). Meaning it will do you more harm than good. It is only the right food combination and preparation that will keep enzymes intact and allow them to be used for the absorption and transportation of all nutrients and substances that cells require.

So, the only possible way of rejuvenating your cells, to look younger, and feel younger and healthier, is by making sure that you provide to the body the right food combination, in order to keep enzymes intact and able to transport all nutrients to the cells.

Food Sources Rich in Enzymes

Enzymes needs to be combined with energy in order to be absorbed efficiently by the body and utilised as combustible by the cells for growth and repair.

The energy sources normally used are Carbohydrate, derived from plant food and Natural Sugars, derived from fresh raw fruit.

All Raw Fresh Fruit & Vegetables

There is nothing better that raw fruits and vegetables, as they are all rich in enzymes. No only they are a good source of protein combined with energy, but by not going through any cooking process it keeps intact their protein and energy contents. The content of energy in these products takes very little time to digest (around 30 minutes). Meaning, cells are receiving all the nutrients and substances efficiently, and you are not overloading your pancreas.

In short, raw fruit and vegetables will do wonders in your face and body. The energy content will make possible the absorption of proteins and all nutrients and substances, and so, your skin will began to restore itself .

This food also makes it much easier to remove waste products produced during the chemical process of digestion. Meaning, you will not suffer from constipation. In fact, it can even stimulate the removal of any toxic element.

All Raw Fresh Fruit, especially the tropical ones such as:

> Coconut, bananas, papaya, pineapple
> kiwi, grapes, figs, avocados
> dates, cranberries, lemons, berries
> mangos, apples, oranges

Rich in enzymes

All Raw Fresh Vegetables, especially the dark green and bright coloured ones like:

> Spinach, broccoli, cucumbers, carrots
> cabbage, peppers, onions, asparagus
> beans, brussel sprouts, radishes, lettuces
> mushrooms, parsley, peas

Rich in enzymes

All Raw seeds and nuts. (not roasted/salted)

Walnuts, hazelnuts, almonds,
sunflower seeds etc

Rich in enzymes

Good sources of proteins combined with carbohydrate

Pulses, nuts, seeds,vegetables, soya products
(soya milk and tofu and soya mince),
cereals (brown rice, organic jumbo oats,
whole grains, and whole wheat products).

Some fruits and vegetables contain the essential amino acids in the right proportion required by the body.

Bananas, Soya, tomatoes, cucumbers,
potatoes, sweet potatoes, carrots, corn,
cabbage, cauliflower, brussel sprouts, okra,
peas, summer squash and kale.

Most of the plant protein does not contain the 8 essentials amino acids in the proportion required by the body. Meaning, they can be low in one of the essential amino acids. For example, grains usually tend to be low in lysine while pulses are short in methionine. But by combining the two together, grains and pulses, you can obtain a high quality enzyme meal.

These shortness's of essential amino acids tend to be different in different protein foods. This means that by combining two different foods, the amino acids of one protein food can compensate for the one lacking in the other (see the groups on next page for the right combination on plant proteins).

Combination of Plant Protein

There are different combinations of plant food proteins that complement one another. The diagram below shows you how to combine plant foods in order to create a high quality protein intake. This is much higher protein quality that the one of meat and dairy products, which are unable to meet energy needs.

Group 1

Grains, Breads and Cereals

Brown rice, wholemeal bread,
whole wheat products
& wholegrain cereals

This includes: all kinds of wholewheat pasta, noodles, wholegrain breakfast cereals and bread, whole flour products , etc. **By combining any item of group 1 above with one single food source from any of the three groups (from the next page), A, B or C, you will obtain the right proportion of the essential amino acids required by the body.** See Table 1 overleaf:

Table1

Group A	Group B	Group C
pulses (legumes)	Vegetables	Nuts & Seeds
Peas, Beans & Lentils	All kinds of veg.	All nuts & seeds
dried beans		Walnuts
Peas, Runner Beans		Almond, Peanuts
Soya, Butter, Kidney Chick peas		Sunflower and others
Split peas, Green peas and others		

Sample Meal of Plant Protein

Red Beans

By combining whole wheat pasta from group 1 with red beans from group A you are obtaining a high quality protein meal. It contains Enzymes, vitamin B, E, C, A, Essential fatty acids and some minerals

Red Beans (200 grams)8.oz	Two carrots
One Onion	One clove of garlic
Herbs	Whole wheat pasta (200 grams) 8.oz
Cashew sauce (page 158)	Virgin olive oil (two tablespoons)

Soak the beans in water for 12 hours. After soaking, rinse well and place in an express pan (Pressure Steamer, this pan cooks a lot faster and it also minimises the amount of nutrients lost) with water, a whole onion, two whole carrots, a clove of garlic, olive oil and some herbs of your choice. Boil all together for around 15 minutes. Cook the pasta in a separate pan. Once is all cooked, serve all together on a plate, cut into pieces the carrots and the onion, and pour this delicious cashew sauce on top. This recipe will serve two people.

You can make all sorts of combinations from Group 1 with group A, B or C such as rice and lentils, butter beans and pasta, rice and vegetables, pasta with vegetable, and so on. By adding some fresh sauces you will obtain a nice and tasty meal. Using this food combination technique, will provide you with a high protein quality meal. Make sure you always use the same method of cooking (soak it for 12 hours and cook in the express pan) for all kinds of beans.

Accompany every single cooked meal with a nice bowl of fresh raw salad (see appendices for some suggestions) of your choice, and take a piece of fruit before and after each meal in order to maximise its nutrients and substances (raw fruit and vegetables are rich in enzymes, vitamins and minerals).

Combination of Protein and Good Fats

Eggs

Eggs are a good source of protein and they contain the 8 essential amino acids in the right proportion required by the body. But only when poached. On the contrary, when hard boiled or scrambled they loose most of the nutrients.   They also contain fatty acids. Meaning it is full of the good fats.

But bear in mind that the good proteins and good fats are all in the yolk. It is advisable not to eat the egg white, if possible.

Fish

Any fish are a good source of protein. As with eggs, fish contain all the essential amino acids on the right proportion. Among all fish, oily fish is another source of Omega 3, full of the good fats (see page 36 for more information on good fats)

Make sure always that these proteins are combined with a bowl of fresh raw vegetable salad of your choice and a piece of fruit before and after meal (full of enzymes, vitamins and minerals) in order to maximise it's efficiency.

Table 2

  Recommended Intakes for Protein, g/day

Age	RDA*	
Women 19 to 49 years	45.0 gr	(1¾.oz)
Women 50+ years	46.5 gr	(1¾.oz)
Men 19 to 49 years	55.5 gr	(2.oz)
Men 50 + years	53.3 gr	(2.oz)

*RDA - Recommended Daily Amount

   Protein intake should not exceed more than twice the RDA shown on this table (for information on the exact amount of grams of protein contained in each food see tables in appendices) .

Chapter2   Good Fats

Good Fats are the second most important nutrient. Even more important than vitamins and minerals. This is because the fatty acids they contain, are really essential to every process of the body and skin.

Essential fatty acids are needed for brain cell function and nervous system activity, hormones, glandular function and immune system. They are also fundamental for the cell wall function. Thus, passing oxygen and nutrients into the cell, and keeping foreign bodies out of the cell i.e. free radicals.

But most of all, they will keep you from developing wrinkles and dehydrated dead skin ! They are the oil that lubricates the skin. These fatty acids not only attract water to dehydrated cells, but they also prevent further loss. So, if you want to say goodbye to all these unwanted lines and dry skin, Omega 3 and Omega 6 is the way to go !. These fatty acids will do wonders.

They will regenerate, soften, and firm your skin. They will also improve your health; you will gain plenty of vitality, and you will lose unwanted fat without going through any weight loss program.

The problem is, that over the past 100 years, there has been an increase in the consumption of Omega 6. This is due to the increasing intake of vegetable oils from corn, sunflower seeds, soya bean and other products available in every corner of the supermarket, but not enough products available containing Omega 3.

Studies have shown that consequently, the ratio in our diet of this essentials fatty acids is off balance (the ratio of n-6 to n-3 fatty acids ranges from 2-3 instead of the traditional range of 1-2) and we need to be consuming more of Omega 3.

It is this off balance ratio of essential fatty acids that is a major cause of skin dehydration and wrinkles. A balanced ratio of these two essential fatty acids is vital for a young look and healthy skin.

Omega 3 also plays an important role in the prevention and treatment of coronary artery disease, hypertension diabetes, arthritis, and other anti-inflammatory and autoimmune disorders and cancer.

Omega 3

Omega 3 fatty acids found particularly in:

> Oily fish such as herring, mackerel, sardines, tuna, salmon and swordfish.

Other base sources of Omega 3 fatty acids are:

> Eggs yolks from both chicken and duck,
> chickpeas, and nuts such as walnuts,
> brazil nuts, hazelnuts and pecans.

Vegetarians must consume Omega 3 from plant sources. These are called ALA's (alpha-linolenic acid) and are found in:

Beans, fruit, flax seed oil and wheat germ. Other sources are lettuce, broccoli, spinach, peas, split peas.

Omega 6 fatty acids

Are found in seed oils such as

> Borage oil, evening primrose oil
> and hemp oil.

Other base sources of Omega 6 fatty acids are:

> Olives, nuts, seeds and seed oils,
> and many vegetables and grains.

Remember that it is the shortness of Omega 3 within our diet that makes off balance the ratio between the two. And so it is highly recommended to eat oily fish four times a week and to take 500mg daily supplement of Omega 3.

Sample meal of Good fats (essential fatty acids) Protein

Mackerel Fines Herbs

It is also rich in Vitamin C, E, A, B, Bioflavonoids, Co-enzyme Q10 and some minerals. Remember that fish is a good source of protein on its own, as it contains all the essential amino acids in the right proportion required by the body. So, combining with other source of protein is only optional.

One whole mackerel or a couple of fillets

Fresh lemon juice

Half cup of fresh parsley

Two boiled potatoes

Spinach (200 grams) 8.oz

Fine herbs

Place the mackerel in the steamer for about 10 minutes. Steam the spinach and the potatoes separately. Blend the parsley with a bit of rice milk until smooth and creamy. Place all onto a plate once is cooked and coat the mackerel with this delicious parsley cream. Garnish it with fresh lemon juice and any fine herbs of your choice. This recipe will serve one person.

Do not forget your piece of fruit before and after the meal and a fresh raw vegetable salad of your choice.

Chapter3   Antioxidants

Antioxidants can be as important as enzymes. This is because antioxidants help the body to produce antioxidant enzymes. The main purpose of antioxidant enzymes is to regulate and repair damage from free radicals.

Lets make it simple ! Free radicals always target the nearest stable molecule, stealing its electron. When the stable molecule loose its electron, this molecule becomes a free radical itself, and consequently, living cells became disrupted.

But antioxidants are powerful anti-ageing nutrients and they do not become free radicals by loosing an electron, (they are stable in either form) but quite the opposite. They stabilize free radicals and flush them out of your system, preventing in this way, cell and tissue damage (caused by free radicals) that could lead eventually to cellular damage, and disease. That was the science bit!

These anti-ageing substances can be found in many food sources, especially in raw food. Remember, all raw food is in its natural state and so, they conserve all of their nutrients. There are plenty of food sources that can be eaten raw, and they have been available for thousands of years. Among them, are some of the vegetables and a delicious range of fruits and nuts. Some of them contain high amounts of antioxidant (for more information see list in appendices) .

Vitamin E

Vitamin E, not only prevents cell damage by disallowing the formation of free radicals, but it can also restore collagen production. Meaning, it can firm loose (saggy) skin.

Among all its properties, vitamin E lubricates and softens dry skin, restores collagen, relieves dryness and itching and promotes circulation. It strengthens the immune system, it is good for healing skin lesions, scar tissues and burns.

If you want to stay young, don't forget your vitamin E! Vitamin E prevents ageing acceleration, repair damaged skin tissue, and restores collagen. Meaning, you will also get younger if you are already getting old. It may also protect against cardiovascular disease and artery clogging plaque-formation.

Deficiency of this vitamin can be responsible for saggy skin, dried skin, wrinkles, hair loss, dandruff, easy bruising and varicose veins.

Food sources rich on Vitamin E

Nuts, spinach, sunflower seeds, asparagus, vegetable oils, such as olive, soy beans, legumes (beans, lentils, split peas, chick peas), brown rice, and dark leafy green vegetables, sweet potatoes and avocados.

Sample meal with Vitamin E

Lentils

It also contain enzymes, Vitamin C,A, B and minerals. Lentils and rice, both are a good source of vitamin E. This combination of brown rice from Group 1 with lentils from group A make it also a high quality protein meal.

Lentils (200 grams)8.oz   Whole Brown rice (a full cup)

Mushroom sauce (see page 157) One whole tomato

One whole onion   One clove of garlic

Herbs   Virgin olive oil (two tbsps)

Soak the lentils in water overnight. After soaking, rinse well and place in an express pan with water, one whole onion, one whole tomato, a clove of garlic, olive oil and some herbs of your choice. Boil all together for around 15 minutes. Place the rice in the steamer and cook for around 10 minutes. Once is all cooked, serve all together on a plate, cut into pieces the onion and garlic, and pour mushroom sauce on top. This recipe will serve two people.

Do not forget to add a bowl of fresh raw salad of your choice and take your fruit before and after the meal.

Vitamin C

Vitamin C, as vitamin E, is another highly active antioxidant and essentially important nutrient. Both of them combat free radical formation, and play a major role in collagen formation (collagen is essential for strength and support to the skin). C and E vitamins are recommended to be taken both together (200 mg of each of them to begin this program, this will facilitate the restoration of your skin complexion).

They stimulate the growth of cells. Due to their antioxidant properties, both vitamins promote the repair of wounds and restore your skin complexion. They also protect your skin from ultra-violet radiation emitted from the sun.

C vitamin is also involved in the control of cholesterol, and is used in the immune system. It fights infections, has anti-viral properties and facilitates the absorption of iron (an important mineral for the function of cells) which is essential for the transportation of oxygen from the lungs to all the body tissues.

So, either if you want to look young, regain your skin complexion, and avoid infections, vitamin C can not be ignored. Symptoms of deficiency among others includes poor skin complexion, saggy skin, tiredness, numerous infections, bleeding gums, loss of muscles, fainting and diarrhea.

All dark green vegetables such as

Spinach, asparagus, green peppers, Brussel
sprouts,broccoli, watercress,
and any other greens. Red and yellow
peppers, tomatoes, cauliflower,
parsley, rose hips and onion are rich in C.

Other food sources rich in Vitamin C

All citric fruits such as oranges,
lemons and grape fruits. Berries,
papaya, pineapple, mangos, avocados,
blackcurrants, kiwi and guava.

Sample of fruit salad with vitamin C

Kiwi & Blackberries

It is also full of Enzymes, vitamin C, A, B, Bioflavonoids
and minerals

Three kiwis   One large mango

Freshly squeezed orange juice   Blackberries (half a cup)

Peel and slice the kiwis into medium pieces. Cut into slices the mango. Mix the fruit gently together with the blackberries into a dessert bowl and pour the fresh orange juice over.

Vitamin A

Vitamin A is the anti-wrinkle nutrient. It will do miracles in your face and body. It prevents drying of the skin, and lubricates and softens even more that vitamin E. It will restore your skin complexion, and lines on your face will minimise.

They also promote and maintain healthy function of your eyes, teeth, gums and hair. So your eyes will start to look healthier, younger and sexier. And you can say good bye to lifeless and dry hair and replace it with a healthy and shiny hair.

As every other antioxidant, Vitamin A prevents the formation of cells that could turn into cancer cells, protects the skin from sun damage, enhances the immune system and resists infections. Deficiency of this vitamin may contributes to the failure of weight loss, ear infection, poor skin complexion, dry skin, wrinkles, unwanted body lines, susceptibility to skin conditions, and dried lifeless hair.

Food sources rich on Vitamin A

Variety of dark orange, red, yellow and green vegetables and fruit such as broccoli, kale, spinach, sweet potatoes, carrots, red and yellow peppers, dark green leafy vegetables, parsley, sweet corn,eggs, liver and fish oil. Apricot, banana, papaya, peach, mango, cantaloupe.

Sample of fruit salad with vitamin A

Banana & Apricot

It is also full of Enzymes, vitamin A, C, B, E, Omega 3 & 6, Bioflavonoids and minerals.

Two bananas   Six apricots

Black grapes (half a cup)   Five cashew nuts

Cut the apricots into pieces and blend it with just enough water to keep going until nice and smooth. Halve the bananas and place on a plate. Pour the apricot cream over and decorate with few halves of grapes and small pieces of cashew nuts.

Bioflavonoids

This chemical is found in fruit and vegetables and it has even more antioxidant power that the vitamin C. It contains anti-inflammatory properties, it promotes cell regeneration, and can repair skin damage and liver damage (mainly caused by alcohol).

They are found in the following food

Apricots, strawberries, green tea, rose hips, broccoli, tomatoes, cherries, red wine, lemons, Grapes, oranges, green peppers, red cabbage, green beans, rhubarb, plums, and blackberries.

Sample of Dessert with Bioflavonoids

Alexandra

It is also rich of enzymes, vitamin C, A, B, E, bioflavonoids and minerals

Two peaches   One apricot

Two nectarines   Twenty Strawberries

One tablespoon of organic honey

Wash and slice the peaches, nectarines and apricot. Place the fruit gently together in a bowl. Blend the strawberries with just enough water to get the process going until nice and creamy. Pour the strawberry cream gently into the fruits and pour over organic honey.

Co-Enzyme Q10

This powerful antioxidant is present in every cell of the body and plays an important role in the production of energy within every single cell. It regulates the oxidation of fats and sugars into energy and is one of the most important nutrients for anyone over the age 30.

It is very beneficial for the skin cells and also in reducing blood pressure and heart rate. CoEnzyme Q10 has been found in high concentrations in healthy hearts. Low levels of this substance may responsible for congestive heart failure.

This substance can be found in a number of foods

Sardines, mackerel, tuna,
salmon, soy oil, spinach and peanuts.

Sample of a meal with Co-enzyme Q10

Sardines

Fish is a good source of protein on its own. This meal contain also Essential fatty acids, vitamin A, C, E, B and some minerals

Two or three fillets   Two chopped tomatoes

of Sardines

(depending on the size)

One chopped onion   Spinach (200 grams) 8.oz

Fresh lemon juice (one tbsp)   Boiled potatoes

Virgin olive oil (one tbsp)

Place the sardines on the steamer with the chopped onion and tomatoes. Steam the spinach and the potatoes each of them on a separate tray. Place all on a plate gently when ready, and season it with fresh lemon juice and virgin olive oil.

You can use a can of sardines instead of fresh fish, if you want to make a fast meal. Many of the sardines available in supermarkets are ok. Make sure they are not smoked ones and always read the label. It should not contain any added ingredients apart from salt and oil.

Add your fresh raw salad to the meal and remember your fruit before and after.

Chapter4   B Complex

B complex, not only plays an important role in the function of a healthy brain and nervous system, but it is the vitamin of beauty.

They are involved in the enzymes reaction within cells and they are vital for healing and promoting new cell growth. They also participate in the metabolism of every single cell of the body. All forms of vitamin B are essential for good eyesight, healthy skin tone, nails and hair.

Vitamin B complex is involved in the metabolism of fats, proteins and carbohydrates, which are essential substances to combat premature ageing and its symptoms, such as saggy and wrinkling skin.

Vitamin B1 Thiamine

It plays an important role in the carbohydrate metabolism and the provision of energy (for all body process). B1 is a vital vitamin for a proper function of the nervous system, muscles and skin complexion.

A deficiency of this vitamin is very likely on a Western diet based on refined food, and the symptoms of deficiency include regular irritability and tiredness, lack of concentration, skin dryness and poor skin complexion.

The prolongation of this deficiency can also lead to a major symptoms such as nervous inflammation (resulting in breathing difficulties, fever and palpitation).

Food sources rich on Vitamin B1

Whole grains, brow rice, brazil nuts, chick peas, kidney beans, lentils, peanuts, soya beans, walnut, wheat germ, yeast, pulses, green vegetables, fish, poached eggs, chicken and turkey.

Vitamin B2 Riboflavin

This one too plays a vital role in the metabolism of carbohydrate. It is also involved in the enzymes reaction within cells, making it essential for healthy skin, nails, hair and good eyesight. B2 vitamin is today the most common deficiency and also very visible. A deficiency causes dermatitis, sore and dry lips and tongue, dry skin and scalp, acne, baldness, ulcers, and in some cases trembling, sleeping problem and nervousness.

Food sources rich on vitamin B2

Asparagus, avocado, broccoli,
brussels sprouts, sunflower seeds,
sprouted seeds, sesame seeds,
wheat bran, wheat germ, whole grains,
brown rice, lentils, eggs, fish and chicken.

Vitamin B3 Niacin

Among their functions, B3 vitamin contributes to the good maintenance of a healthy blood and circulation, the nervous system and the function of the adrenal gland. Thus, vital functions for a healthy skin tone (and for your brain). Deficiency of this vitamin causes saggy skin, but also irritability, sleep problem, depression, headaches and tiredness.

Remember that depression, and sleeping problems are a form of free radical and one of the reasons for ageing acceleration.

Food sources rich on B3

Beans, peanuts, almonds, brown rice,
rice bran, sesame seeds, sunflower seeds,
wheat bran, wheat germ, tomatoes,
carrots, fish and chicken.

Vitamin B5 Panthothenic acid

It is involved in the metabolism of carbohydrates and fats, in the maintenance of the immune system and in the function of the adrenal glands. Deficiency of this vitamin is not as common as it is with the others. But when it happens, the symptoms are similar to those deficiency symptoms of the other B vitamins such as headaches and sleeping problems. It may also be responsible for poor adrenal gland function, and abdominal pain.

Food sources rich on B5

Almonds, peanuts, yeast, legumes,
mushrooms, wheat germ, wheat bran,
sesame seeds and eggs.

Vitamin B6 Piroxidine

As many other B vitamins, B6 is involved too in the proper metabolism of carbohydrates and fats, which are fundamental for a healthy skin tone. It also takes part in the manufacture of red blood cells and in the proper functioning of the immune system. Deficiency of this vitamin can result in arteriosclerosis.

Food sources rich on B6

Bananas, beans, yeast, wheat germ, wheat bran, sesame seeds, brown rice, soy beans, corn, hazelnut, walnuts, broccoli, carrots, lentils and tuna.

Vitamin B9 Folic Acid

Apart from being vital for the correct metabolism of carbohydrates, fats and proteins and for the production of blood cells -all indispensable for a young skin complex - it is also responsible for the correct functioning of vitamin B12. A deficiency on this vitamin is very common and the general symptoms are irritability, depression, anaemia, tiredness, and loss of memory.

Food sources rich on Folic acid

> Legumes, green leafy vegetables,
> mushrooms, sprouted seeds, soy beans,
> oranges, almonds, yeast, brown rice,
> wholegrain, salmon, tuna and chicken.

Vitamin B12

While folic acid is vital for the correct functioning of B12, vitamin B12, is vital for the correct functioning of folic acid. As many other B vitamins, B12 is also vital in the metabolism of carbohydrates, fats and proteins, and in the production of blood cells. It is as well very important in the production of nucleic acids, in the maintenance of healthy cells and in the normal functioning of the brain. In other words, it is important in many of the process that contributes to a healthy and young skin.

Deficiency is very common, and evidence has shown that this is due more to bad absorption of the vitamin, than to a lack of the vitamin in the diet. The most common symptom is anaemia. However, a prolonged deficiency can cause severe depression, sleep disturbance, lack of coordination, irritability, loss of certain reflexes and speech coordination.

Food sources rich on B12

Yeast, cauliflower, eggs, herring, leafy greens, liver, mackerel, tuna, salmon, mushrooms, and spirulina.

PABA-Para-Amino-Benzoic Acid

It helps to synthetise folic acid and assists on the break down of proteins. A deficiency is may be one of the reasons for eczema and in many cases for grey hair

Food sources rich on PABA

Yeast, nuts, beans and all kind of legumes, sardines, mackerel, tuna, leafy greens, spinach, herring, wholegrain, oats and wheat germ.

A sample of soup that covers all the B vitamins

Traditional Soup

It contain also Enzymes, vitamin B, E,C, A, Omega 6 and some minerals

Half cup of brown rice   One carrot

Two leeks   Two tomatoes (med. size)

Ten Mushrooms   Shredded sorrel

Sesame seeds (two tablespoons)

Wash all the vegetables and chop into pieces. Cook the carrots and leeks in the steamer. Steam the rice in a separate tray and once cooked, place it into the blender. Add to the blender the steamed carrots and leeks, and the fresh tomatoes and mushrooms. Blend it all together until smooth. Garnish it with the shredded sorrel and sprinkle some sesame seeds. This soup should serve one person.

Do remember always your piece of fruit before and after every meal and a bowl of raw fresh salad to go within each meal.

B Supplements

It is recommended to take a daily B complex supplements (one capsule per day) to maximise the efficiency of the food with B vitamin content and to compensate for the loss of nutrients of cooked food.

A good B complex supplement should look like this:

Table 3

Thiamine (B1)	50mg
Riboflavin (B2)	50mg
Niacin (B3)	50mg
Pantothenic Acid (B5)	50mg
Vitamin (B6)	50mg
Folic Acid	500 ug
Vitamin B12	50 ug
PABA	50mg

Make sure that B1, B2, B3, B5 and B6 always contain the same amount (25 mg to 50 mg is the right amount).

Chapter5 Minerals

Vitamins and substances do miracles. But they will only work efficiently with the presence of minerals. Minerals play a vital role in almost every single reaction that takes place within our cells. They are essential for the function of many enzymes and they are involved in the metabolic process. Minerals are also vital for a healthy brain function and a good bone structure.

In other words, vitamins, enzymes and good fats require the presence of minerals in order to function correctly. Minerals are as vital as every other substances for the maintenance of an optimum skin and health condition. So if your aim is for a rejuvenated face and body, including minerals in your diet is the way to succeed.

Minerals are required in small amounts, but the damage caused by the deficiency can be very visible and serious. They are as important as every other nutrients - already mentioned - which you simply can not ignore.

All these minerals can be obtained from eating a varied diet. There is plenty of fresh food available in the market that contain all the nutrients that the body requires. It is important to take a daily (one capsule per day) supplement of multivitamins & minerals in order to reinforce the lower amount of nutrients from cooked food.

Remember that supplements are not food. They are only a reinforcement to your daily food intake, and they won't work if you ignore eating all the right things (see Part 3 for life style and adjustments).

Selenium

Selenium keeps the skin elastic, and believe it or not, most people have a deficiency of this powerful antioxidant. It is vital for the activity of some enzymes and for a proper functioning of the liver and blood system. It protects your heart and improve your circulation.

Food sources rich in selenium

Grapes, garlic, onions, egg yolk, yeast, carrots, oranges, cabbage, almonds, brazil nuts and pecans.

Sample of Selenium mix

Grapes & Almonds

It contain Enzymes, Essential fatty acids, Vitamin C, B, E, minerals and Bioflavonoid

Grapes (a full cup)   Almonds (around ten)

Plain and simple dessert full of selenium and deliciously tasteful. Wash the grapes and place it on a bowl. Blend the almonds with enough water to produce a milk and pour it gently on to the grapes.

Zinc

It is indispensable for a great skin and so it is for a strong and shiny hair. This is because of its participation in the function of many enzymes during the metabolic process and its contribution with vitamin A utilisation, which role, among many others is to protect and lubricate the skin, to enhance the immune system and resist infections, and promotes the healing of wounds.

Food sources rich in zinc

Spinach, lettuce, carrots, cucumbers, barley, brazil nuts, almonds, walnuts, and hazelnuts, chicken, eggs, fish, legumes, olives, sardines, soya beans, soy lecithin.

Sample of meal rich in Zinc

Poached egg

Eggs are a good source of protein on its own. This meal contain also essential fatty acids, vitamin A, C, B and Bioflavonoids, selenium, calcium and other minerals.

Two medium eggs	One chopped pepper
Few slices of truffle	Onion sauce (see page 157)

Break the eggs and place them in a pan with hot water. Poach for about 3 minutes. Once ready, serve on a plate with the slices of truffle. Add the chopped pepper and spread around the onion sauce.

Magnesium

As with many of the minerals, this one too is essential for the correct function of many enzymes during the metabolic process. Involved in the utilisation of vitamins B1 and B12, it contributes to a good bone structure and firmness of your skin and as well as your teeth. Deficiency causes anxiety, muscle tremor, chronic fatigue and muscle pain and deficiency is very common in today's diet. You loose magnesium and calcium by eating too much chocolate! And remember, it won't do any favours to your skin and neither to your hair.

Food sources rich in Magnesium

Seeds, soya beans, leafy green vegetables, apples, apricots, avocados, bananas, peaches, brown rice, lentils, fish, oats, almonds, peanuts, pistachio, sesame seeds, wheat germ, whole grains.

Sample of breakfast full of Magnesium

Oats

This breakfast contain as well enzymes, Omega 6, vitamin E, C, A, B, Bioflavonoids and some other minerals

Half cup of organic oats	One full cup of soya milk
Fresh lemon juice	Sesame seeds (two tblsp)
One banana	One apple

Boil the oats with the soya milk. Cut the banana and apple in slices. Place all in a bowl, add the seeds, and pour over one tablespoon of fresh lemon juice

Calcium

Calcium, as the same as magnesium, is vital for a good bone structure, firmness of your skin and strong teeth and hair. This is because calcium is essential for growth and repair. Calcium and magnesium work in balance in a ratio of 2:1 and loosing the ratio is one of the reasons for low energy feeling and fatigue. But it will not make a difference how adequate your intake of calcium is within your diet, if you eat a lot of sugar and table salt. It just won't work. All minerals and vitamins in general are affected by salt and sugar.

Food sources rich in calcium

> Fish (especially oily ones) soya milk, almonds, soya beans, leafy green vegetables, sesame seeds, asparagus, bananas, brazil nuts, hazelnuts, cabbage, broccoli, olives, sunflower seeds

Sample of breakfast rich in calcium

Muesli

It also contain enzymes, Omega 3, vitamin E, C, A, B and other minerals

½ cup of organic muesli One full cup of soya or rice milk

20 grams (¾.oz) of brazil nuts and hazel nuts

A handful of fresh fruit such as cherries and cranberries.

Place the muesli on a dessert bowl, add gently the cherries and cranberries. Spread the nuts and pour the milk over.

Boron

Boron is another vital mineral for your skin and well-being. It participates in the utilisation of calcium (which is essential to the skin and bones) in the activity of vitamin D and in the balance of oestrogen and progesterone.

Food sources rich in Boron

Grapes, apples, pears and spinach

Sample of a fruit dessert with Boron

Pears and Apples Delight

It also contain Enzymes, omega 3, vitamin E, B, A and some other minerals

Two pears   Two apples

Ten Walnuts

Halve the pears and apples. Blend the walnuts with a bit of your favourite milk to make a delicious cream. Arrange the pears and apples in a plate and pour the walnut cream over the fruit.

Chromium

It is essential in various metabolic activities such as the utilisation of fats and sugars, glucose and insulin tolerance and in the function of the immune system. A lack of this mineral can be responsible for depression, irritability and sleeping problems.

Food sources rich in chromium

Whole food and fresh fruit

Sample of a dessert with chromium

Strawberries Delight

This tasteful delight contains also Enzymes, Omega 3 and 6, Vitamin C, B, E, A, Bioflavonoids and other minerals

Twenty strawberries   Half a cup of raspberries

Pineapple (100 grams)4.oz   Pistachios (around 10)

Wash all fruit. Blend the raspberries with a bit of water until smooth. Cut the pineapple and strawberries into slices and mix together in a plate. Pure the raspberries cream over and sprinkle with chopped pistachios.

Iodine

Iodine is vital for a firm young skin complexion. It is also essential for the regulation of metabolism and growth. This mineral is necessary for the proper function of the thyroid gland and so to keep your body weight regulated. Deficiency may causes enlargement of the thyroid gland, weight gain, and tiredness.

Food sources rich in Iodine

All leafy green vegetables, asparagus, blueberries,strawberries, watermelon, garlic, cucumber, mushrooms, peanuts, sesameseeds, soya beans,spinach, seaweed, seafood and other fresh fruits.

Sample of vegetable salad with Iodine

Prawn salad

It is also rich in Enzymes and it contains Omega 3 and 6, vitamin E, C, A, B, Bioflavonoids and some other minerals

Three Leafs of lettuce	Five asparagus
Two medium size tomatoes	One onion
Virgin olive oil (two tablespoons)	Prawns(a full cup)
Five slices of cucumber	

Plain and simple salad rich of iodine and easy to make. Cut all vegetables in pieces after a good wash. Chop the onion and place all together in a bowl. Add the prawns and season it all with olive oil.

You can substitute prawns for any other seafood of your choice (they all contain iodine). Have some fun finding your own favourite combinations.

Manganese

A good skin tone definitely needs this mineral. Manganese it is not only indispensable for the activity of many enzymes and metabolic reactions, which are essential for a young and healthy skin, but it is also involved in the nerve and muscle functions. It is implicated in the growth and health of the skeleton which are responsible for the maintenance of a proper bone structure, including the one in your face. Deficiency of this mineral could lead to rheumatoid arthritis.

Food sources rich in Manganese

Nuts, whole grains, avocados, pulses and tea

Sample of cocktail rich in Manganese

Avocados & Nuts

This cocktail it contains also enzymes, Omega 3 and 6, vitamin E, C, B, A and other minerals

Ten almonds   Five hazelnuts

Five Cashews   Two avocados

Try a nice and simple snack cocktail. Peel the avocados and cut it into medium slices. Place in a bowl and spread the nuts around.

Potassium

Potassium is a fundamental ingredient of cell and tissue fluids, that contribute to the water balance of your skin and it is also vital for nerve function. So if your skin is dry, you are probably lacking in this mineral. An off balance ratio of potassium/sodium can be very common on today's diet. Although potassium levels are quite high in many whole foods, they are quite often low in the highly processed ones.

Deficiency symptoms in potassium include weakness of muscles, sickness, pins and needles, low blood pressure and headaches.

Food sources rich in Potassium

Bananas, papaya, avocados, apricots, dates, raisins, carrots, sunflower seeds, brazil nuts, hazelnuts, brown rice, chick peas, lentils, parsley, sesame seeds, soya beans, wheat germ, wholegrain, garlic, almonds.

Sample of cocktail with Potassium

Banana & Nuts

It also contains enzymes, Omega 3 and 6, vitamin E, A, B and some other minerals

One banana   Dates (half a cup)

Ten Brazil nuts   Sesame seeds (two tblsp)

Peel the banana, cut it into small pieces and place gently in a bowl. Spread the brazil nuts and dates, and sprinkle all with some nice sesame seeds.

Iron

Iron is a vital component for the transportation of oxygen (an essential element for cells to stay alive) to all the cells and so it is for your skin. Iron can be enhanced if it is taken with vitamin C. Deficiency of iron causes anaemia, with symptoms of shortness of breath, swelling ankles, feeling cold. Pregnant women and those who have just given birth are also at risk of iron deficiency.

Food sources rich in Iron

Egg yolk, nuts, green vegetables, apricots, avocados, brown rice, chick peas, lentils, kidney beans, soya beans, sunflower seeds, Parsley, peaches, pears, raisins, and pulses.

Sample of a sauce rich in Iron

Genoise Sauce

This delicious sauce it contains also enzymes, Omega 3 and 6, vitamin C, A, B, bioflavonoids and some other minerals

Herbs	Half a cup of pistachios
Half a cup of almonds	Two yolk of eggs
Two tablespoon of lemon	Pepper
Olive oil (two tablespoons)	

Blend the pistachios and almonds with your favourite herbs and enough water to produce a milk. Whisk with the yolks of eggs until completely smooth. Season with lemon juice and pepper and finish with organic or unrefined virgin olive oil.

Use this tasteful sauce with fish, any kind of beans or with any other meal of your choice.

Sulphur

Sulphur is essential for the proper metabolism, for the manufacture of proteins and for the production of collagen. In other words, sulphur is vital for your bones, skin, teeth and nails. It keeps the skin elastic, it cleans the blood and tissue of toxic build up and it is involved in human longevity. With sulphur you will look and feel younger. You will be provided with a lot of energy and you will feel far more healthy than ever before.

Food sources rich in Sulphur

Raw onions, garlic, asparagus, broccoli, red pepper, hemp seeds, pulses and fish

Sample of salad rich in sulphur

Cendrillon Salad

It also contains enzymes, Omega 6, vitamin E, C, A,B, and other minerals

Three med. boiled potatoes	One red pepper
Two long pcs. celeriac	One truffle
Five asparagus tips	One artichoke
Mushroom sauce (see page 157)	One onion or viniagarete

Make sure that the potatoes are cooked in the steamer in order to loose the least nutrients and taste as possible. Wash well all the vegetables, cut them into small pieces and place gently on a plate. Season with mushroom sauce or vinaigrette.

PART 2

How You Are Accelerating Your Ageing Process

Chapter6   Free Radicals in Food

We all are quite aware of how unfriendly free radicals can be to our skin and our well-being. When a free radical enters your body it destroys the molecules, causing cells to die prematurely and affecting the other living cells left.

Let me give you one example. Collagen molecules provide strength and support to the skin. If a free radical attacks these molecules, it will break the link between them and as a consequence you will end up with a fragile skin structure.

Our body is programmed to battle and minimise free radicals, and our food intake is the indispensable combustible used by cells in order to succeed. The problem is that instead of providing the combustible, "nutrients and substances" in order to combat free radicals, all you are doing is confronting your body with an extra provision of free radicals - those encountered in your wrong daily food and drink intake -.

So, what it is that you are doing wrong with your food intake, that is making you to deteriorate and age faster than you are supposed to ? Some people probably eat too little of the good food. While others eat a reasonable amount of the good food but they are combining with the wrong ones. There are various ways of preparing and combining food that cause major free radicals to form.

Among those are; the processed food, refined food and bad fats.

These preparations and/or combinations, change the structure of food; alter their molecules and destroy their proteins and substances, making cells unable to receive any nutrients from them.

It is the lack of nutrients encountered in many of these foods, and consequently, the difficulties with the digestion process, the main factors why you are ageing before time.

So, it does not matter how much you try to avoid every other free radicals, (which is a good thing), or how many creams and expensive treatments you try to put on your face and body (creams and expensive treatments don't regenerate or repair your skin. Neither they prevent early ageing. They just hide the problem, and only on a temporary basis), because until you decide to avoid all the free radicals that you are including daily in your food and drink intake, you will be ageing before time.

The good news is that you can reverse all of these symptoms and prevent any further ones. Avoiding all these bad foods and following a proper diet, will transform your look.

You will regain muscle tone. Your skin will go firmer and your eyes will regain their structure, making your expression to look much younger. You won't have to worry any more about skin dehydration and dry hair (see part 3 for life style adjustments).

Chapter7   Processed Food

Any food that goes through a process is called processed food. Among all the processing techniques, one of them is cooking. Cooked food, either home-made or not, causes free radicals to form.

Temperatures above 105 degrees C. alter the food molecules, and so also their proteins, nutrients and substances. So, you can imagine what happens to the food when you start to expose it above this temperature. Baking, frying, grilling, barbecuing and microwaving, involve temperatures of 120-160 degrees C.

Meaning, there is little nutrients left if any, in food once exposed to these levels of temperature. One study found that microwaving reduced the amount of antioxidants in some foods by 97% and boiling by 66%. - On the contrary, with a steamer, nutrients are reduced by only 11% - .

Neither are there many enzymes left once food is cooked in any of these ways. Enzymes or proteins, are a very fragile substance and these high temperatures destroy most of them. As there are little enzymes and nutrients left in these foods, you could almost say that, apart from probably gaining few extra pounds in your body, you are just eating for nothing.

And is not only your skin cells that are suffering by preventing the body from receiving the proteins and nutrients they required.

Your pancreas will end up overloaded and exhausted after so much work in digesting food which lacks nutrients and substances. As the pancreas is linked to the liver function, you could also get liver problems. And you already know what liver problems can do ! It will certainly give you bags under your eyes and your skin may turn a shade of yellow.

These foods, sooner than later, will make you feel tired, with lack of energy and poor concentration (chronic fatigue is caused mainly by the ingestion of food low of proteins and nutrients and is a very common symptom in our Western diet). In other words, your body is degenerating and ageing faster that it is supposed to.

But food exposed above 105 degrees C. temperature is not the only processed food that you are consuming daily.

There are other techniques of food processing quite common on today's diet. Among them:

Fermentation, emulsification, addition of gas for bread and drinks, pasteurization for dairy products, packaging, mixing, deep frying and spray drying).

As with all the cooking processes, these processing techniques alter the food molecules too, and also the food structure and their nutrients and substances.

You probably do not realise that many of the products that you normally store in your fridge freezer and comes in a box, can, bag or carton has been processed (and/or refined) up to some extent by one of these methods. And some of them probably by more than one method.

This can include fast food or ready meals, soft drinks, and other high calorie products.

Normally the ready meals have usually been cooked in the oven, grill or frying pan. Meaning, these foods have already being exposed to temperatures above 105 degrees C. and are left with little protein and nutrients. They normally recommend on the carton box instructions to reheat in the microwave or oven. So it will be exposed to high temperature not once, but twice.

Processed foods can also be added with salt, sugar, and some chemicals. They are added for various purposes, such as adding colour, stabilizing, preserving, sweetening, thickening, softening, adding flavour etc.

Many of these chemical compounds can not be assimilated properly throughout the digestion process as they are unknown to the human body and some of them may be toxic to humans.

And it is not only your skin that suffers from these compounds. Although side effects vary from person to person, many symptoms have been reported. Among them; drowsiness, tingling, headache, burning sensation, facial pressure or tightness, nausea, etc.

So, not only are you destroying indispensable nutrients from your food throughout the cooking process, but you are also buying food which are already low in nutrients in the first place and with additives.

Believe it or not, to the human body, all these ways of preparing and cooking food are very recent. For millions of years, the human diet has been based on fruits, nuts, vegetables, grains and seeds. And our body is well adapted to deal with these types of food and get nutrients out of them.

Our body is not adapted to take care of food with low amounts of enzymes and nutrients. And this is another reason why you are ageing before time. Even if you consume a reasonable amount of fresh and healthy food, it will almost be for nothing when you combine it with processed food.

What is the point of having steamed vegetables, or making a nice and fresh raw salad, if you go and add some chips with it and probably some processed salad dressing or any other processed sauce on top ?

Although it is still better to eat some good food than none, by combining a healthy raw salad or steamed vegetables with fried potatoes and/or processed salad dressing, you are minimising the efficiency of nutrients and enzymes contained in the vegetables.

Chips, as any other fried food are exposed to temperature above 105 degreesC. and there are little enzymes and nutrients left in the potatoes after this cooking process.

This also occurs with processed salad dressing. As it is not fresh dressing, it must contain some kind of additive. These additives alter the food molecules and structure and so then their nutrients and substances.

Consequently, these kind of foods interfere with the absorption and transportation of proteins and nutrients to the bloodstream.

Meaning, cells won't be able to receive all enzymes and nutrients provided with your salad and/or steamed vegetables. And your pancreas will also have to work harder in order to digest this fried food and/or processed salad dressing.

There is only one way to go, if you want to look young and healthy, and that is by avoiding any product that has been exposed and/or requires temperatures above 105 degrees C. during the cooking process.

There is a extensive range of fresh ingredients available in the supermarket. Try to buy them and make your own salads, sauces, soups and juices with it. When you cook, make sure you use the steamer.

Avoid any food or drink already made (see part 3 for life style adjustments). Make sure you always read the label when you buy some of them and eliminate from your diet those that contains chemical additives. There are some products in cans that are ok, such as oily fish and many different kinds of beans. Canned beans are normally boiled in a commercial sized pressure steamer with water and salt. As long as you remove the water and rinse them well, they should be ok. The same goes for all the oily fish. These fish are normally cooked in pressure steamers with added oil and salt. Avoid any other added ingredient that is not oil or salt.

Chapter8   Refined Food

Among all the refined foods, anything made of white flour is refined and so it is with our Western diet of white flour, white bread, white sugar, white rice, white pastry, white pasta, processed oil, margarine, refined juices, bakery products etc.

Most of the refined foods lack vitamins, minerals and fibre. This is because most of the nutrient elements as well as the bran and fibre, are situated on the outer layers of the grain. And when wheat or any other grain is refined, the outer layer is removed.

They tend to remove or separate the outer layer of the grain in these foods, in order to prevent it from going rancid and to make it to last longer on the supermarket shelf.

Many of these products have added salt, sugar, preservatives and are highly acid forming. These additions are made with the purpose of preserving and returning some taste to the food   -once the outer layer of the grain and its nutrients are removed, food is left with little taste-

As a result of the refining process, food is left with low amounts of nutrients and some of them with additives.

This is just another way of preventing your cells from receiving all the essential nutrients and substances. Instead, you harm your cells with a diet which is high in fat, salt, sugar, preservatives, which are highly acid forming and highly refined. You overload your pancreas after the hard work involved within the digestion process.

The removal of the fibre in all flour products has been blamed for constipation that affects so many of us today. When food remains in the colon, eventually it begins to putrefy. Meaning, that germs could eventually invade the food and start to rot within us, all this results in the production of toxic wastes.

It is only a matter of time before all this toxic waste can reach the bloodstream and travel to every single part of the body and so every cell can be affected.

This toxic waste could harm your nervous system and make you depressed and irritable. It could also harm your digestive organs, so you end up bloated and distressed with gas. And if it is doing all this to your health, you can imagine what is doing to your face and body, much before you see any of these problems.

Painful varicose veins and heaviness around your eyes, are among the most common symptoms. Your skin will go shallow, saggy and wrinkled. Neither your hair will get away with it; and it will go thinner and thinner.

So, just remember, that this toxic waste, plus the fact that you are preventing your cells from receiving the nutrients and substances they require to combat and minimise cell destruction, and the addition of chemical compounds in these foods, it will surely make you age and degenerate much before time.

Carbohydrate, bran and fibre are essential to the body, but certainly, few of the nutrients are in white flour products.

Swap all white flour products for the brown ones. Substitute white rice for brown rice and white bread for brown wholemeal (see chapter 3 for more information). Use all the wholemeal products such as whole wheat and wholegrain for pasta and cereals instead of white ones.

The Dorian Gray Diet

Chapter9   Bad Fats

We all need to eat fat as part of are diet, as it is essential to the body and to the skin. Probably even more essential than vitamins and minerals. But there is a difference between Good Fats and Bad Fats.

The Good Fats includes Omega 3 and Omega 6 fatty acids (for more information on good fats go to chapter 2) while the saturated fats are the Bat Fats and includes meat and dairy products.

Many of these Bad Fats products have also been processed and/or refined, and some others have also been pasteurised. Saturated fats (Bad Fats) are found mainly in animal products such as:

Red meat

Butter, lard, and some margarines

All Cheeses, particularly hard cheese,

Milk (especially the full fat one)

Fatty meats and meat products such as sausages and pies,

You can also find these animal contents in some products such as:

Cream, soured cream and ice cream

Some snacks such as crisps

Biscuits, cakes and pastries

Sweets and chocolates.

Meat and dairy products (see chapter 1 for more information) are not a good source of protein. Protein can only be efficient when combined with energy such as a carbohydrate (from plants) and natural sugars (from fruits).

Excessive eating of these products can also block the basement membrane. This basement consist on a filter between small blood vessels and cells. When the basement is blocked, nutrients and oxygen can not pass through quickly and efficiently from the blood into the cell which is where they are needed.

And the same occurs with waste products. Waste products of cell metabolism needs to pass out of the cell quickly in order to avoid poisoning the interior of the cell. When the membranes are blocked, some waste product will remain within your cells.

So you can imagine all the harm caused to the cells by the consumption of these products. Bad fats deprive cells from receiving the nutrients and oxygen they require.

Instead, the body is left with too much waste product that harms the interior of the cells.

And If it is doing this to your cells, never mind what it is doing to your face and body. Droopy and dry skin, bags under your eyes, varicose veins and many other unwanted problems.

High consumption of these products has also being associated with hormonal problems, osteoporosis and in some cases cancer. It does also produce an imbalance ratio between calcium and magnesium, which are essential minerals for the skin. It may also increase bad cholesterol in your blood.

And guest what ! This bad fats are very likely to make you gain too much weight. This is because bad fats contain only small quantities of fatty acids (which is the fats needed by the body). So, your body won't be satisfied enough and will keep asking you constantly for more food until it manages to receive the full amount of fatty acids required.

This is another benefit of following this program. So not only will you look younger and feel healthier and happier, but you will loose all the unwanted fat in your body without going into any a weight loss program (see part 3 for life style adjustments).

PART 3

Action Plan

Instructions And Adjustments
Towards Rejuvenation

It is only now that you have learned the reasons why you are ageing faster than you are supposed to, that you can begin to rectify and rejuvenate yourself. This programme will show you step by step how to succeed.

Our body is depending on the consumption of the right food; food full of nutrients and substances. All these foods will provide you with an energy that you haven't experienced for many years. It will decrease the speed at which you are ageing and it will repair the skin tissues that have already been damaged.

So you won't have to worry any longer about wrinkles and other imperfections around your face and body, once you start to follow this program.

Some of you will probably find it a sacrifice to start with. But it all depends of how you want to see it. If you think carefully, the majority of people spend a total of 2 hours daily of pleasure (time taken eating between 3 to 4 meals a day) consuming the wrong food.

In return, they get 8 hours of poor sleep with all the consequences (including ageing), 14 hours of discontent, anguish and distress (for being forced to live with an unwanted degenerated and wrinkled body and face or undergoing painful treatments which don't solve the problem as it only lasts a few months) and physical discomfort and a feeling of heaviness (as soon as you reach age 35 or 40) together with a lack of vitality. This can lead later to numerous and successive illnesses.

I don't know about you, but I decided to choose 22 hours of happiness and 2 hours of sacrifice !.

The *positive* part of this program is that within two weeks you will get used to this change of habit and your new diet won't be a sacrifice any longer. You will start to taste and enjoy all the nice and healthy varieties of fresh food.

From the third week onwards, you will begin to experience a rejuvenation process taking place in your skin, and also inside your body. Your body and face will stop deteriorating any further. You will notice your body start to go much lighter and active and you will regain the vitality that you haven't experienced for many years.

You will sleep much better (deep sleep contributes noticeably to cell rejuvenation) and you will become a much more positive and a happier person.

Your skin will start to regain muscle tone and gradually, within time, all those unwanted lines around your face will fade.

A healthy liver will provide you with a more firm and plain stomach, a firmer skin around your eyes, and a healthier skin colour.

PART 3

Chapter10   Life Style Adjustments

What to do in 24 Steps - For Success

Step One

Make sure you eat plenty of raw fruit and vegetables

Ensure that all your cooked meals are accompanied with a big bowl of fresh raw salad in the same quantity as your main meal, and eat your fresh raw fruit before and after every meal. Remember that nutrients and substances in raw foods are always intact (as they haven't been exposed to heat by any cooking process) and so, it will compensate and maximise the efficiency of your cooked meal. You can have as many raw vegetables and fruits as you want. Use them as an snack too.

Remember that raw food is rich in enzymes and enzymes is what you need in order to allow the absorption and transportation of all nutrients to the cells.

Step Two

Add fish to your diet

Swap meat products for fish, especially for oily fish, such as mackerel, sardines, salmon, tuna and herring among others. They all contain the good fats and they all do goodness to the skin, hair and body. Make sure they are always cooked in the steamer. You can also buy in tins. Most of them are ok, as they have been cooked in steamers. But always read the label for the ingredients and choose those which contain no other additives apart from oil (preferable olive oil) and a small amount of salt.

Step Three

Add eggs to your diet

Eggs (only the yolk, avoid the white content) contain the good fats too, and they are a good source of protein in its own right. Ideal for the skin and heart. Try a couple of egg yolks every other day of the week, or you can have it every day. Make sure you have it poached. When cooked in other ways such as hard boiled, fried or scrambled they loose vitamins and nutrients and it will do more harm that good to you.

Step Four

Add all kind of nuts and seeds to your diet

They are all full of vitamins, good fats, proteins and minerals. Some of them are high in calories but you don't need more than 30g per day. You can use seeds and nuts as snacks, or you can mix them with your cereals breakfast and/or meals. Make sure you choose the ones with no added salt. Too much salt can be detrimental to the skin and your health.

Step Five

Avoid all Food containing Saturated Fat and Hydrogenated Oil

Bad fats are not giving you any favours. They deprive your cells from essential nutrients and destroy the proteins within your body.

Avoid red meat, fatty meats (such as sausages and pies) lard, and all full fat dairy products such as butter, some margarines, full fat cheese and milk. Bad fats are also encountered in some snacks and crisps, cream, soured cream, ice cream, biscuits, cakes, pastries, sweets and chocolates.

If you are a meat eater, try not to consume meat more that 3 times a week. Choose lamb or white meat such as chicken, turkey and/or any other poultry products instead of red and fatty ones. And make sure at least, that the meat you are buying is fresh (remember that processed meat contain preservatives and additives).

Replace full cream milk for soya milk (soya is a high quality protein on its own) or rice milk. But make sure that you read the label to ensure that it contains added calcium.

Replace margarine for unrefined raw oils to spread on your bread (such as borage oil, extra virgin olive oil, evening primrose oil and hemp oil). Otherwise use butter which still better than margarine. But remember that it contains saturated fat, so try to avoid it as much as you can.

Step Six

Eliminate all frying, grilling, barbecuing, microwaving and baking

These methods of cooking are a source of the largest amount of free radicals. The high temperature to which the food is exposed (120-160 degrees C.) destroys all proteins and nutrients from food making it difficult to digest and causing body degeneration.

This includes cakes biscuits, pastries, snacks and so on. Anything that it has been cooked in one of these ways will degenerate your body a lot faster than you think.

Step Seven

Try to use the steamer as much as possible

The amount of nutrients lost by cooking in a steamer are a lot lower than cooking in any other ways (it reduces the amount of nutrients by only 11%). Use the steamer as much as possible for vegetables that requires cooking, fish and other foods. Remember that baking, grilling, frying and microwaving create the most free radicals and one of easiest way of speeding up your ageing process.

Step Eight

Avoid Sugar .

You can not stay young if you keep eating sugar. Excess of sugar alters the protein's function and consequently, it will alters your cells too. It also alters the balance between calcium and phosphorous. Meaning, you will loose the firmness of your skin and end up with a saggy and wrinkled face and body as a consequence. It does not matter how many supplements of minerals you decide to ingest, if you keep consuming sugar, it will all be for nothing. Lack of calcium can also result in osteoporosis later on in life.

Avoid sugar in your drinks and all sugar products, such as cakes, biscuits, puddings, cereals and so on.

The best way of replacing sugar is consuming a lot of fresh fruit, as they contain natural sugars, and are essential to the body as a source of energy during your digestion process. After few days, fruit will be sweet enough for you and your sugar craving will be for fruit instead of cakes and biscuits (a spoon of natural honey can be added to help you with craving). Replace sugared cereals for a nice organic rolled oats.

However, if you eat occasionally some sort of sweet (once or twice a week as a treat), make sure that you keep taking plenty of fruit.

Step Nine

Avoid added Salt products and stick to the daily amount required.

High amounts of salt draws calcium from your bones which is excreted in your urine. Excessive consumption of salt can be detrimental to your health and so to your skin. It is best not to eat more that 2.4 grams per day. For best results, read the label of every single products that you buy in the supermarket and choose those with no added salt or with the lowers amount of it as possible (you only have to do this once). Count the total amount of salt within the products you are consuming and try to meet most of your daily intake recommended with an organic table salt on a nice bowl of fresh salad or with your favourite meal.

Step Ten

Avoid all Processed Food

This kind of food has a minimum of nutrients and is usually high in salt, sugar, bad fats and preservatives. Many of the instant food prepack products that come in a box, can, bag and carton are processed food. This includes many cereals, meat, potatoes, bread, smoked food, pickled and salted products, sweet sour, sauces, mayonnaise, salad cream, tomato sauce, some prepack salads, baked products etc.

It is highly recommended to eat fresh meals, but if you decide to buy occasionally any of the ready prepared meals, make sure you read the labels in advance. Some of the foods that come in tins, can be ok, such as all kind of organic beans (make sure you remove the water that comes in the tin and rinse the beans before consuming) and all varieties of oily fish.

Step Eleven

Avoid all Refined Foods and swap them   for Whole products instead

Every product made of white flour is refined. Avoid all of them. Choose always wholegrain products (the first ingredient should be whole such as wholegrain, whole wheat, wholemeal or whatever type of bread you choose) instead of white bread. Eat brown rice instead of white rice, whole wheat pasta instead of white pasta and organic rolled oats, instead of any other oats. Go for unrefined oils (they should say unrefined on the label) and fresh and natural juices made by yourself from the fruit itself. For the occasionally treat, find some bakery product made with brown sugar or honey (avoid refined honey, go for the natural raw instead) and brown flour.

Step Twelve

Make your own sauces and juices

Try your own sauces and juices with fresh raw ingredients and avoid all the processed and refined ones with preservatives and sugar. Start to enjoy the taste of real food and nutrients and rejuvenate yourself with these natural juices and sauces full of enzymes.

Step Thirteen

Avoid Pasteurised Products

All pasteurised products such as milk, yoghurt, cheese, etc. contribute to ageing acceleration. Not only do they contain bad fats, but they all are exposed to 160 degrees of heat or more during the pasteurisation process. This high temperature diminishes the vitamin's content and it changes the milk protein to an inorganic form which can not be assimilated by the body. Thus, making the body unable to digest and so, preventing your cells from receiving nutrients.

Try to avoid all pasteurised products. Replace cows milk for soya and/or rice milk. Both of them contain proteins, calcium, vitamins and minerals and are very beneficial to your skin and health.

Step Fourteen

Avoid eating too much Chocolate

Even by consuming chocolate with no added sugar, the body still looses the ratio balance between calcium and magnesium. These minerals are vital for the structure and firmness of the skin, and also for teeth and hair.

Chronic fatigue is caused as well by lack of magnesium and it is a symptom of degeneration.

If you eat chocolate or any other kind of sweets once or twice a week, make sure you still eat plenty of fruit.

Step Fifteen

Avoid Re-heating food

The more often you expose to heat your food, the more nutrients it will loose and the more you will be overloading your pancreas during the digestion process. Make sure at least, that your meal is not going to be exposed to heat more than once. Sometimes it can look very convenient to reheat cooked food from previous day, but it is not doing any favours to your skin and body.

Step Sixteen

Reduce the amount of coffee and tea intake

The body looses 45 mg of calcium per each three cups of coffee. If you find it difficult to stop drinking coffee, replace it with decaffeinated, and do not exceed more than two cups a day.

Bear in mind too, that coffee, tea and every other hot drink has been exposed to high temperatures and so, they will destroy the enzymes (as you already know, enzymes are very delicate substances and susceptible to heat) from your body, including the enzymes from the food that you have consumed just previously to your intake of coffee, or any other hot drink.

So, we recommend that you reduce the number of hot drinks to the minimum. Make sure there is a gap of at least an hour before and after your meals, between any hot drink consumption and don't reheat your drinks in the microwave.

Tea is a good source of antioxidants although contains caffeine as well. Avoid drinking too much of it and try to replace it with green tea, mineral water, soya milk, rice milk and natural fruit and/or vegetable juices.

Steep Seventeen

Avoid all Fizzy drinks

The consumption of fizzy drinks may lead to cellulite and flaccid and saggy skin in face and body (even some teenagers are already having these kinds of symptoms). According to scientific research, (in the public domain) these kind of drinks may make you old before time. The high amount of phosphates that some of them can contain was found to make the skin and muscles wither and could also damage the heart and kidneys.

Remember as well that the amount of sugar and chemical content in some of these products, destroy proteins from the body. Eating the right food will have no effect, if you continue consuming these type of drinks - no fizzy drinks – period.

Step Eighteen

Avoid any other Processed drinks

Many drinks that come in a bottle or carton, have been processed to some extent and can be detrimental to the skin and your health. Many of them contain some kind of artificial ingredient and some others are full of added sugar and preservatives. This also includes the traditional instant hot drinks such as hot chocolate, that are supposed to relax you before you go to sleep, when in reality many of them are supplying you with a mixture of additives that will not let you sleep at all.

Avoid the consumption of all of them and replace with fresh, natural fruit and vegetable juices, green tea, soya milk and rice milk.

Step Nineteen

Keep alcohol consumption to the minimum

A little bit of alcohol is allowed on this program, but only in moderation (2 units, twice a week) and it should not be taken as part of a daily routine.

Believe me!, 14 units per week for women and 21 units for men as recommended in the UK may harm your liver, and consequently this will inflame your eyelids. You may get bags under your eyes and your skin may turn a shade of yellow, and of course, dehydration and wrinkles are yours for 'free'.

Drinking two units of alcohol daily will prevent your body from absorbing all the essential minerals and nutrients required by your cells for the formation and maintenance of the skin and bones. It has been demonstrated by scientists that chronic drinkers suffer from bone deterioration.

Choose an organic wine (no added sulphates) instead of a big cocktail of chemicals contained in some spirit drinks. Organic red wine is full of antioxidants and drinking in such a moderation, it could probably do more good than harm to your health.

Step Twenty

Don't over drink water

Water is a basic and essential element for our body. But drinking too much of it can be detrimental to your health and also to your skin.

All food contains water and if you follow this program, you will be consuming food that contains a large amount of the water required by the body.

The human body consists of 80% of water. So eating food that is rich in water such as fruit and vegetables, should almost meet the amount of water that your body requires.

So it is not a necessity to drink two litres of water daily in order to prevent dehydration and/or to detox your body. In fact, the over consumption of water (or any other drinks such as coffee, tea and fizzy) could wash out a good deal of the nutrients in your body, including the fatty acids which are so essential to the skin. And that's what definitely will make your skin dehydrated !.

The best recommendation is to listen to your body, and drink water only when you feel thirsty and not otherwise (except on exceptional circumstances such as very hot weather or fever).

Step Twenty One

Avoid the consumption of any food or drink at extreme temperature.

Remember that proteins (enzymes) are very fragile substances and that exposing food to high temperatures, destroys all their enzymes. But eating and drinking products at extreme temperature (either too cold or too hot) will also destroy the enzymes contained in your body. Remember that without enzymes, your digestive tract becomes unable to absorb nutrients and you will age a lot faster than you would like.

Make sure that you wait a few minutes for your cooked meal and/or hot drink to cool down before you eat or drink it. But most of all, try to avoid the consumption of hot and cold drinks and food as much as possible. Make sure you consume all your drinks at room temperature.

Even raw fresh fruit (which is full of enzymes) is difficult to digest when cold. Make sure that you take it out of the fridge at least one hour before consumption.

Avoid the consumption of ice creams and cold cakes in your diet. This can be detrimental to your health due to the extreme temperature and the amount of sugar content.

Step Twenty Two

Avoid any type of artificial sweetener

Any artificial sweetener is not natural. They are unnatural as they are processed derivatives of food and/or chemicals. Meaning they are difficult to digest and it may harm the enzymes stored in your body. Choose natural sweeteners or stevia (a natural sweet herb) instead of the artificial ones.

Step Twenty Three

Make sure you sleep your hours

Make sure you sleep between 8 and 9 hours every night. A good nights sleep plays an important role in cell rejuvenation. Remember that sleep deprivation is another big factor of ageing acceleration. Sleeping difficulties are due most of the time to a poor diet and the chemical compounds in food and drinks.   By following this program your sleeping difficulties will become history and is not only your face that will notice it, but you will also feel a much calmer and happier person.

Step Twenty Four

Stop Smoking

While some people can stop smoking at once, others need to do it in a gradual way. Even if it takes you a year to quit smoking, start right now. The good news is that you will find much easier to stop smoking by following this program. This is because nicotine craving is much higher after eating fried and all sorts of processed and saturated fat food.

It is recommended to take vitamin C supplements while you are still smoking .

Appendices

Recipes & Eating Suggestions

There are lots of nice fresh foods that you can eat. Here are some recipes and suggestions. Many others will come to your imagination once you have started. And believe me ! Once your start to discover the real delicious taste of food, you won't want to eat anything made from artificial ingredients and low in nutrients! Because real food contains nutrients, it gives the real taste and pleasure of eating and makes you feel good and look great.

And remember! Food low in nutrients make you constantly hungry. You can never get satisfied enough and you then have to keep eating more and more of the wrong low nutrient food.

Kitchen Tools

Real food requires only three essential kitchen appliances. These are: steamer, express pan (pressure steamer) and a blender.

The steamer should be used for all vegetables that require cooking, potatoes, fish and meat. Very little nutrients (11% only) are lost by this way of cooking. For all kind of beans and lentils always use the express pan. It cooks a lot faster (15 minutes) and it looses less nutrients that boiling.

Remember that the purpose of eating is to grow young and healthy. So you can start to get rid of now from your kitchen all those nasty appliances that are making you old, tired, heavy and unhappy.

The blender will introduce you to all the nice and tasteful sauces, soups, cocktails and desserts. Say good bye to your oven, grill, frying pan, microwave and start a new life from today.

Breakfast Recipes

Oats

This breakfast contains enzymes, Omega 6, vitamin E, C, A, B, bioflavonoids and minerals

Half cup of oats	One full cup of soya milk
Fresh lemon juice	Sesame seeds (two tblsp)
One banana	One apple

Boil the oats with soya milk. Cut the banana and apple into slices and place in a bowl with the oats. Add the seeds, and pour over the fresh lemon juice.

Poached Eggs (yolk only)

Just a simple breakfast that will provide you with enzymes, Omega 3 and 6, vitamin E, C, A,B and some minerals

2 fresh eggs

2 slices of wholegrain bread

1 tablespoon of organic or unrefined virgin olive oil

Choose your favourite vegetables such chopped onion and three pieces of lettuce cut in slices to maximise the efficiency of this cooked protein.

Poach the eggs only in the minimum time in order to be able to digest it properly. Once it is poached, place the egg yolks on a plate and add the vegetables. Spread the olive oil on the bread. Ignore the egg white – discard.

Muesli

Rich in enzymes, Omega 3, vitamin E, C, A, B and some minerals

½ cup of organic muesli

One full cup of soya milk or rice milk

20 grams (¾.oz) of brazil nuts and hazel nuts

A handful of fresh fruit such as cherries and cranberries.

Place the muesli in a dessert bowl, add gently the cherries and cranberries. Spread the nuts and pour the milk over.

Light Meals Compound salads

Allemande Salad

This salad contain enzymes, Omega 3, vitamin E,C,A,B and minerals

Two half apples,

Chopped parsley and onions

Two steamed potatoes, (cooled down)

Fillets of herrings (steamed)

Half cup of diced gherkins,

Ten thin slices of beetroot.

Vinaigrette sauce

Wash all fruit and vegetables. Halve the raw apples and the steamed potatoes, and put together on a plate. Add the gherkins and the herring fillets, and decorate with the slices of beetroot. Spread over the chopped onions and parsley. Season with vinaigrette sauce (a mix of water, lemon juice, salt, vinegar and unrefined or organic olive oil).

No fresh herrings? , replace with tinned ensuring no additives are present.

Andalouse Salad

It contains enzymes, Omega 6, vitamin E,C,A, B, bioflavonoids and minerals

Half cup of whole grain brown rice

Crushed garlic(one teaspoon)

1 Chopped onion

Chopped parsley

One tablespoon of apple cider vinegar

Two or three tomatoes

Two tablespoon of olive oil

Sweet pimentos/sweet peppers (10 slices)

Black pepper

Steam the rice. Wash the tomatoes and pimentos. Cut each tomato in four pieces and place around the rice with very thin slices of sweet pimento. Crush the garlic and spread it around together with the chopped onions and parsley. Season with organic or unrefined virgin olive oil and organic cider vinegar and sprinkle on a bit of black pepper.

Imperial Salad

It contains enzymes, Omega 6, vitamin E, C,A, B, Bioflavonoids and minerals

A full cup of French beans,

Two Carrots,

One apple

Chopped parsley

One truffle

Parsley sauce

1 tablespoon of fresh lemon juice

Cook the beans in the steamer. Wash the apples and truffles, cut them in very thing slices and place around the beans. Grate the carrots on top, chop the parsley and spread over. Season with parsley sauce and fresh lemon juice.

Cendrillon Salad

It contains Enzymes, Omega 6, vitamin E, C, A,B and minerals

Three medium sized steamed potatoes

One red pepper

Two long pieces of celeriac

One truffle

Five asparagus tips

One artichoke

Mushroom sauce (see page 157) or vinaigrette

One onion

Make sure that the potatoes and artichoke are cooked in the steamer in order to loose the least nutrients and taste as possible. For the other vegetables, cut them into small pieces and place gently on a plate. Add the potatoes and artichoke and season all with mushroom sauce or vinaigrette.

Bagatelle Salad

It contains enzymes, Omega 6, vitamin E, C, A, B and minerals

Two carrots

Five asparagus tips

One full cup of mushrooms

Organic virgin oil (one tablespoon)

Plain and simple salad but a delicious one too. You can just add it to any meal or simply have as a snack. Just wash well all the vegetables and cut the mushrooms and carrots into a very thin slices. Add the asparagus tips and dress with your favourite sauce or with organic virgin olive oil.

Prawn salad

This tasteful salad contains Enzymes, Omega 3 and 6, Vitamin C, B, E, A, Bioflavonoids and mineral

Three leafs of lettuce

Five asparagus shoots

Two medium size tomatoes

One onion

Virgin olive oil (two tablespoons)

Prawns (a full cup)

Five slices of cucumber

A delicious salad rich in iodine and easy to make. Cut all vegetables in pieces after a good wash. Chop the onion and place all together in a bowl. Add the prawns and season it all with olive oil.

You can substitute prawns for any other seafood of your choice (they all contain iodine). Have some fun finding your own favorite combinations for all salads. Add some different oils of your choice such as; borage oil, sunflower oil, evening primrose oil and hemp oil. They all taste delicious and are a good source of Omega 6.

The Dorian Gray Diet

Sauces

Genoise Sauce

This delicious sauce contains enzymes, Omega 3 and 6, vitamin C, A, B, bioflavonoids and minerals

Herbs

Half a cup of pistachios

Half a cup of almonds

Two yolk of eggs

Two tablespoon of lemon

Pepper

Two tablespoons of virgin live oil

Blend the pistachios and almonds with your favorite herbs and enough water to produce a milk. Whisk with the yolks of eggs until completely smooth. Season with lemon juice and pepper and finish with organic or unrefined virgin olive oil.

Onion Sauce

This simple and tasteful sauce contains enzymes, Omega 3 and 6, vitamin E, C, B,A, Bioflavonoids and minerals

Two onions (medium size)

Half a cup of Soya milk

nutmeg

Salt (1 gram) pinch

Pepper

Strain and chop the onions. Blend one chopped onion with soya milk and make a sauce. Add the other chopped onion on top of the sauce and season with salt, pepper and nutmeg.

Cucumber Sauce

This sauce is rich of enzymes Omega 3 an6, vitamin E, C, A, B and minerals

Half a cucumber (unpeeled)

Four tomatoes

Peeled almonds (around ten)

One garlic clove

Black pepper

Wash all the vegetables and chop them. Blend the almonds with enough water to produce a milk. Then add the vegetables, garlic and spices and blend again until smooth.

Mushroom Sauce

Taste delicious and is rich of enzymes, Omega 3 and 6, vitamin C, B and minerals

Fifteen mushrooms

One tablespoon of freshly boiled/steamed barley

Half cup of walnuts

One tablespoon of fresh lemon juice

Two cloves of garlic

Wash the mushrooms and leave to dry. Chop the mushrooms and garlic. Blend all the ingredients together with half a cup of water to make a smooth and delicious thick cream.

Cashew Sauce

It contains enzymes, Omega 3 and 6, vitamin C, A, B and minerals

Half a cup of cashews

One chopped onion

Dried parsley

Half a green pepper (chopped)

Rice milk

Blend the cashews with rice milk. Use a little less milk for a thick cream and more milk for a more pouring one. Add the rest of the ingredients and blend again until completely smooth and thick.

Soups

Tomato Soup

It is rich of enzymes, Omega 6, vitamin C, E, A and minerals

Ten tomatoes

Cumin powder

Black pepper

Dried parsley

Half a cup of sago

Few lettuces chopped in small pieces

Boil the sago in water. Chop the tomatoes in quarters and put in to the blender (with no added water). Add the cumin powder, pepper and parsley and blend once more until completely smooth . Add some water after and blend it again if you desire a little less thick soup. Finally, pour the soup in a bowl and place the sago and the chopped lettuce on top.

Cream of Green Peas Soup

Rich on Omega 6, vitamin A and minerals

| Half a cup of fresh peas | Barley flour |
| One carrot | Five mushrooms |

Wash well all vegetables and cook in the steamer (placing each vegetable in a separate section). Blend the peas with barley flour and some water. For a thinner soup just use a little more water. Simmer for 10 minutes. Garnish the soup with the boiled dices of carrot and mushrooms.

Traditional Soup

It contain Enzymes, vitamin B,E,C, A, Omega 6 and minerals

Half cup of brown rice   One carrot

Two leeks   Two tomatoes

Ten Mushrooms

Shredded sorrel

Sesame seeds (two tablespoons)

Wash all the vegetables and chop into pieces. Cook the carrots and leeks in the steamer. Steam the rice in a separate tray and once cooked place into the blender. Add to the blender the steamed carrots and leeks, and the fresh and raw tomatoes and mushrooms. Blend all together until smooth. Garnish with the shredded sorrel and sprinkle some sesame seeds. This soup should serve one person.

Cream of Pumpkins Soup

It contains enzymes, Omega 6, vitamin E, C, A, B, bioflavonoids and minerals.

Pumpkin (100grams) 4.oz   Two onions

Two leeks   Dried parsley

Two tablespoons of fresh lemon juice

Chop the leeks and onions. Boil the leeks in the steamer. Place the boiled leeks and raw onions into the blender with a bit of fresh water to start the blending process. Blend until smooth and place in a bowl. Remove the skin from the pumpkin, then wash, steam it and blend it with a bit of rice milk until nice and creamy. Pour the pumpkin cream into the soup and garnish it with dried parsley and fresh lemon juice.

Cream of swede Soup

Rich in Enzymes, Omega 6, vitamin C, A and minerals.

Swedes (200 grams) 8.oz   Black pepper

Beetroot (ten thin slices)   Dried parsley

Remove the skin from the swede, chop it into small
pieces, wash it, and cook in the steamer. Place the swede
into the blender with a bit of soya milk until smooth.
Pour it into a soup bowl and garnish it with thin slices of
beetroot, black pepper and parsley.

Cocktail snacks

Banana & Nuts

Rich in potassium. It also contains enzymes, Omega 3 and 6, vitamin E, A, B and some other minerals.

One banana	Dates (half a cup)
Ten Brazil nuts	Sesame seeds (two tablespoons)

Peel the banana, cut it into small pieces and place it gently in a bowl. Spread the brazil nuts and dates, and sprinkle all with some nice sesame seeds.

Avocados & Nuts

Rich in manganese. It also contain Enzymes, Omega 3 and 6, vitamin E,C,B, A and other minerals

Ten almonds   Five hazelnuts

Five Cashews   Two avocados

Try a nice and simple snack cocktail. Peel the avocados and cut into medium slices. Place in a bowl and spread the nuts around.

Main Courses

Main Courses

You can make all sorts of combinations from Group 1 with group A, B or C (see chapter 1 for groups) such as rice and lentils, butter beans and pasta, rice and vegetables, pasta with vegetable etc. Add some fresh sauce and you will obtain a nice tasteful meal. Using this food combination technique, will provide you with a high protein quality meal. Make sure you always use the same method of cooking (soak it for 12 hours and cook it in the express pan) for all kinds of beans and lentils.

Accompany every single cooked meal with a nice bowl of fresh raw salad of your choice, and take a piece of fruit before and after each meal in order to maximise its nutrients and substances (raw fruit and vegetables are rich in enzymes, vitamins and minerals).

Fresh Cod Fish

Remember that fish is a good source of protein on its own as it contains all the essential amino acids in the right proportion required by the body. So combining with any other source of protein is optional. This meal is also rich in enzymes, Vitamin C, E, A, B, Omega 6, Bioflavonoids, and minerals

One portion of fresh cod fish	Fresh chopped parsley
Plain boiled potatoes	Half a cup of green peas
Barley flour	Lemon juice

Wash the fish well and place in the steamer for about 10 minutes or until cooked. Steam the green peas and blend with the barley flour. Add a bit of water to make a nice and smooth sauce.

Simmer the peas and barley blend for 5 minutes. Place the fish and the boiled potatoes onto a plate. Pour the green peas sauce on top and garnish it with fresh lemon juice and chopped parsley. Accompany every single cooked meal with a nice bowl of fresh raw salad of your choice, and take a piece of fruit before and after each meal in order to maximise its nutrients and substances (raw fruit and vegetables are rich in enzymes, vitamins and minerals).

Fresh Salmon

This fish is a good source of (Good fats) protein by itself. This meal is also rich in enzymes, Essential fatty acids, vitamin C, E, A, B, Co-enzyme Q10 and minerals

One portion of fresh salmon   Cucumber sauce (p156)

Whole brown rice (half cup)   Four slices of truffles

Place a thick slice of salmon in the steamer after a good wash and steam for about 15 or 20 minutes (check it occasionally as time varies pending on the size of the fish). Place the salmon into a plate and coat with cucumber sauce. Serve with boiled brown rice and garnish with slices of truffles.

Accompany every single cooked meal with a nice bowl of fresh raw salad of your choice, and take a piece of fruit before and after each meal in order to maximise its nutrients and substances (raw fruit and vegetables are rich in enzymes, vitamins and minerals).

Mackerel Fines Herbs

This fish is a good source of (Good fats) protein by itself. This meal is also rich in enzymes, Essential fatty acids, Vitamin C, E, A, B, Bioflavonoids, Co-enzyme Q10 and some minerals.

One whole mackerel or a couple of fillets

Fresh lemon juice

Half cup of fresh parsley

Two medium size boiled potatoes

Spinach (200 grams) 8.oz

Fine herbs

Place the mackerel in the steamer for about 10 minutes. Steam the spinach and the potatoes separately. Blend the parsley with a bit of rice milk until smooth and creamy. Place all onto a plate once cooked and coat the mackerel with this delicious parsley cream. Garnish with fresh lemon juice and any fine herbs of your choice. This recipe will serves one person.

Accompany every single cooked meal with a nice bowl of fresh raw salad of your choice, and take a piece of fruit before and after each meal in order to maximise its nutrients and substances (raw fruit and vegetables are rich in enzymes, vitamins and minerals).

Fresh Herring

Another good source of (Good fat) protein on it's own. A meal rich in enzymes, vitamin E, C, A, B, Omega 3 and 6, bioflavonoids, Co-enzyme Q10 and minerals

One whole fish

Fennel (100 gr) 4.oz

Brown rice (half cup)

Chopped mushrooms (100 gr) 4.oz

Parsley sauce (p177)

Fresh lemon juice

Wash well the fish, split and bone it. Place in the steamer for about 10 minutes until cooked. Steam the fennel on a separate tray after a good wash. Serve the fish and fennel with boiled brown rice and garnish with the chopped mushrooms, fresh lemon juice and parsley sauce.

Accompany every single cooked meal with a nice bowl of fresh raw salad of your choice, and take a piece of fruit before and after each meal in order to maximise its nutrients and substances (raw fruit and vegetables are rich in enzymes, vitamins and minerals).

Fresh Haddock

A good source of protein on it's own. A meal rich in Enzymes, vitamin E, C, A, B, Bioflavonoids, Omega 3 and 6, and minerals

One fillet of haddock

Genoise sauce (see page 154)

Chopped parsley

Green peas (a full cup)

Plain boiled potatoes

Steam the haddock after a good wash and also the potatoes and green peas, (all in a separate trays). Once cooked, place all on a plate, sprinkle the haddock with chopped parsley and garnish it with genoise sauce.

Accompany every single cooked meal with a nice bowl of fresh raw salad of your choice, and take a piece of fruit before and after each meal in order to maximise its nutrients and substances (raw fruit and vegetables are rich in enzymes, vitamins and minerals).

Red Beans

By combining whole wheat pasta from group 1 with red beans from group A you are obtaining a high quality protein meal.. It contains Enzymes, Omega 6, vitamin B, E, C, A , Essential fatty acids and minerals

Red Beans (200 grams)   8.oz

Two carrots

One clove of garlic

Herbs

Whole wheat pasta (two full cups)

Cashew sauce (page 158)

Virgin olive oil (two tablespoons)

One whole onion

Soak the beans in water for 12 hours. After soaking, rinse well and place it in an express pan (this pressure steamer pan cooks a lot faster and it also minimises the amount of nutrient lost) with water, a whole onion, two whole carrots, a clove of garlic, olive oil and some herbs of your choice. Boil all together for around 15 minutes. Cook the pasta in a separate pan. Once all cooked, serve all together on a plate, cut into pieces the carrots and the onion, and pour the delicious cashew sauce on top. This recipe will serve two people.

Lentils

Lentils and rice, both are a good source of vitamin E. This combination of brown rice from Group 1 with lentils from group A make it also a high quality protein meal. It also contains Enzymes, Omega 6, Vitamin C,A, B, Bioflavonoids and minerals

Lentils (200 grams) 8.oz

Brown rice (a full cup)

Mushroom sauce (see page 157)

One whole tomato

One whole onion

One clove of garlic

Herbs and Virgin olive oil (two tablespoons)

Soak the lentils in water overnight. After soaking, rinse well and place in an express pan with water, one whole onion, one whole tomato, a clove of garlic, olive oil, and some herbs of your choice. Steam all together for around 15 minutes. Boil the rice. Once is all cooked, serve all together on a plate, cut into pieces the onion and garlic, and pour the mushroom sauce on top. This recipe will serve two people.

Sardines

Fish is a good source of protein by itself. This meal contain also Essential fatty acids, vitamin A, C, E, B, Omega 3 and 6, Co-enzyme Q10 and some minerals

Two or three fillets of sardines (depending on the size)

Two chopped tomatoes

One chopped onion

Spinach (200 grams)8.oz

Lemon juice (one tablespoon)

Boiled potatoes

Virgin olive oil (one tablespoon)

Place the sardines on the steamer with the chopped onion and tomatoes. Steam the spinach and the potatoes, each of them on a separate tray. Place all on a plate gently once ready, and season it with lemon and olive oil. You can use a can of sardines instead of fresh fish, if you want to make a fast meal. Many of the sardines available in supermarkets are quite safe. Make sure they are not smoked ones and always read the label for signs of additives.

Accompany every single cooked meal with a nice bowl of fresh raw salad of your choice, and take a piece of fruit before and after each meal in order to maximise its nutrients and substances (raw fruit and vegetables are rich in enzymes, vitamins and minerals).

Poached egg

Eggs are a good source of protein by itself. This meal contain also Essential fatty acids, vitamin A, C,B and Bioflavonoids, selenium, calcium and other minerals.

Two medium eggs   Pepper

Few slices of truffle   Onion sauce (see page 155)

Break the eggs and place them on a pan with hot water. Poach for about 2 or 3 minutes. Once ready, serve on a plate with the slices of truffle. Add some pepper and spread around the onion sauce.

Accompany every single cooked meal with a nice bowl of fresh raw salad of your choice, and take a piece of fruit before and after each meal in order to maximise its nutrients and substances (raw fruit and vegetables are rich in enzymes, vitamins and minerals).

Lamb pasta

This meal is rich in vitamin C, E,A,B, Bioflavonoids, Omega 6, and minerals

Mince lamb (200 grams)	Chopped garlic (two cloves)
Whole wheat pasta (full cup)	Chopped tomato (two)
Chopped parsley	Herbs
One chopped red pepper	One chopped green pepper
Genoise sauce (page 154)	Olive oil (one tablespoon)

Wash the meat well before, if you mince it yourself, and steam it together with the chopped garlic, tomato, herbs, parsley and red pepper, for about 15 minutes or until cooked. Serve it on the plate with the pasta and mix well with a tablespoon of olive oil. Sprinkle the chopped green pepper around and pour the Genoise sauce or any other sauce of your choice.

Accompany every single cooked meal with a nice bowl of fresh raw salad of your choice, and take a piece of fruit before and after each meal in order to maximise its nutrients and substances (raw fruit and vegetables are rich in enzymes, vitamins and minerals).

Chicken

This meal is rich in vitamin C, E,A,B, Omega 3 and 6, Bioflavonoids and minerals

Two pcs of chicken (200grams) 8.oz   One courgette

Chopped tomato (two med. Ones)   One chopped onion

Garlic powder   Dried parsley

Mushroom sauce (page 157)   Fresh lemon juice

Plain boiled potatoes

Coat the chicken with two tablespoons of fresh lemon juice. Add garlic powder on top and place it in the steamer together with the chopped tomatoes and chopped onion. Steam the courgette and potatoes on separate trays. Serve all on a plate, sprinkle the dried parsley and pour over the mushroom sauce or any other sauce of your choice.

Accompany every single cooked meal with a nice bowl of fresh raw salad of your choice, and take a piece of fruit before and after each meal in order to maximise its nutrients and substances (raw fruit and vegetables are rich in enzymes, vitamins and minerals).

Desserts

Alexandra

Rich of Enzymes, vitamin A, C, B, E, bioflavonoids and minerals

Two peaches

One apricot

Two nectarines

Twenty Strawberries

One tablespoon of organic honey

Wash and slice the peaches, nectarines and apricot. Place the fruit gently together in a bowl. Blend the strawberries with just enough water to get the process going until nice and creamy. Pour the strawberry cream gently onto the fruit and spread the organic honey.

Cardinal

Rich of Enzymes, vitamin A, C, B, E, bioflavonoids, Omega 3 and 6 and minerals

Ten strawberries   Two peaches

One pear   Raspberries (100grams) 4.oz

Five walnuts

Wash all the fruits and place the raspberries into a blender with a bit of water and blend until nice and smooth. Cut the strawberries, pear and peaches into small pieces. Mix all the fruit together and pour the raspberries puree over it. Decorate with walnuts cut in small little pieces.

Pears and Apples Delight

It contains   Enzymes, Omega 3, vitamin E, B,A and minerals.

Two pears

Two apples

Twenty Walnuts

Halve the pears and apples. Blend the walnuts with a bit of your favourite milk to make a delicious cream. Arrange the pears and apples on a plate and pour the walnut cream over the fruit.

Banana & Apricot

It is full of Enzymes, vitamin E, C, B, A, Omega 3 and 6, bioflavonoids and minerals

Two bananas   Six apricots

Black grapes   Cashew nuts

Cut the apricots into pieces and blend with just enough water to keep it going until nice and smooth. Halve the bananas and place on a plate. Pour the apricot cream over and decorate with few halves of grapes and cashew nuts.

Strawberries Delight

This tasteful delight contains Enzymes, Omega 3 and 6, Vitamin C, E, B, A, Bioflavonoids and Minerals

Twenty strawberries   Half a cup of raspberries

Pineapple (100 grams) 4.oz   Pistachios (around 10)

Wash all fruit. Blend the raspberries with a bit of water until smooth. Cut the pineapple and strawberries into slices and mix together on a plate. Pour the raspberry cream over and sprinkle with chopped pistachios.

kiwi & Blackberries

It is full of Enzymes, vitamin C, A, B, Bioflavonoids and minerals

Three kiwis

One large mango

Freshly squeezed orange juice

Blackberries (half a cup)

Peel and slice the kiwis into medium pieces. Cut into slices the mango. Mix the fruit gently together into a dessert bowl with the blackberries and pour the fresh orange juice over it.

Grapes & Almonds

It contain Enzymes, Essential fatty acids, Vitamin C, B, E, minerals and Bioflavonoid

Grapes (a full cup)

Almonds (around ten)

Plain and simple dessert full of selenium and deliciously tasteful. Wash the grapes and place in a bowl. Blend the almonds with enough water to produce a milk and pour gently onto the grapes.

Desserts

Best Foods That Are Enzyme Rich

How to Plan Your Meals

You can use the recipes listed on the appendices as a starting point. All of the recipes are well balanced in protein and carbohydrate. See the table below for the daily recommended amount of protein intake, do not exceed the Recommended Daily Amount (RDA) more that twice. Make sure that 40% of your daily food intake is based on carbohydrates.

You can also have some fun combining food of your own choice (see all the tables for the amount of grams on protein and carbohydrate contained in every single food) and the three groups combination for plant protein.

Imperial Conversions

1 gr/g/gramme	= 1/25 Ounce	
12.5g	= ½ Ounce	
25g	= 1 Ounce	
100g	= 4 Ounces	¼lb
200g	= 8 Ounces	½lb

Don't be *too* exact with your weighing – life's too short!

Recommended Intakes for Protein, g/day

Age	RDA*	
Women 19 to 49 years	45.0 gr	(1¾.oz)
Women 50+ years	46.5 gr	(1¾.oz)
Men 19 to 49 years	55.5 gr	(2.oz)
Men 50 + years	53.3 gr	(2.oz)

*RDA - Recommended Daily Amount

Protein intake should not exceed more than twice the RDA shown on this table for information on the exact amount of grams of protein contained in each food see later on in this chapter.

Combination of Plant protein

Grains, Breads and Cereals

Brown rice, bread, Whole wheat products & Wholegrain cereals. This includes: all kinds of pasta, noodles, breakfast cereals, flour products, wheat products, etc.

By combining any item above with one single food source from any of the three groups below, A, B or C, you will obtain the right proportion of the essential amino acids required by the body.

Group A	Group B	Group C
pulses (legumes)	Vegetables	Nuts & Seeds
Peas, Beans & Lentils	All kinds of veg.	All nuts & seeds
dried beans		Walnuts
Peas, Runner Beans		Almond, Peanuts
Soya, Butter, Kidney Chick peas		Sunflower and other seeds
Split peas, Green peas		

Plant Food Protein & Carbohydrate in Grams

Group 1

Bread, Cereals and Grain	Protein	Carbohydrate
Brown rice (100g)	4.4g	23g
Oats (Wholegrain 100g)	13.5g	58.7g
Wholemeal bread (100g)	15.9g	29.8g
Wholemeal rolls (100g)	8.9g	30g
Pasta wholewheat (100g boiled)	13g	65g
Wheat-Durum (100g)	14g	70g
Wheat-Hard Red (100g)	15g	68g
Wheat-Hard White (100g)	11g	76g

Group A

Protein & Carbohydrate in legumes. Peas, Beans & Lentils (100 grams) with no added salt. (cooked in express pan)

Legume	Protein	Carbohydrate
Butter beans	5.5 g	19g
Beansprout	6g	19g
Kidney beans	6.5g	20g
Runner beans	6g	19g
Chick Peas	7.5g	19g
Lentils	9g	15.5g
Green peas	8g	21g
Soy beans	7g	15g
Split peas	10g	41g

Group B

Protein & Carbohydrate in vegetables (100 grams) with no added salt. (Steamed)

Vegetable	Protein	Carbohydrate
Artichoke	4.47g	3g
Asparagus	4g	3g
Aubergine	2g	2.5g
Beetroot	2.7g	9g
Broccoli	3.5g	2.5g
Brussel Sprouts	4g	5g
Cabbage	2g	5g
Carrot	1.6g	9g
Cauliflower	4g	4.1g
Celery	2.2g	2g
Chicory	1.2g	4g
Courgette	3.2g	3g
Cucumber (with skin)	1g	1.3
Fennel	1.2g	2.3g

Group B Continued	Protein	Carbohydrate
French beans	11.4g	2.5g
Gherkins	1.2g	3g
Gourd	1.5g	2g
Leek	1.7g	4g
Lettuce (raw)	0.8g	1.5g
Lima beans	13g	16g
Mushrooms	2g	1g
Okra	2.4g	3.5g
Olives	1.2g	3.8g
Onion (cooked)	0.8g	8g
Onion (raw)	2.5g	16g
Spring onion (raw)	2g	7g
Parsnip	1.5g	14g
Peas	8g	12-15g
Peppers (raw)	1g	2g
Potatoes	1.6g	15-25g
Pumpkin	0.7g	3g
Radish	0.7g	3g
Red Bell Pepper (raw)	1g	2g
Soya (milk)	7.8g	0.2g

Group B Continued	Protein	Carbohydrate
Spinach	2g	1.8g
Squash summer	1.9g	2g
Swede	0.6g	6g
Sweet potatoes	1.8g	15-20g
Sweetcorn	2.6g	3g
Spirulina (dried seaweed	60g	16g
Tomatoes (raw)	2g	3g
Turnip	0.8g	5g
Watercress (raw)	3g	0.5g
Yam	2g	28g

Group C

Protein & Carbohydrate in Nuts & Seeds with no added salt .(per 100g)

	Protein	Carbohydrate
Almonds	21g	7g
Amaranth	4g	50g
Barley	3g	28g
Brazil Nuts)	16g	3g
Cashews	23g	23g
Flax seeds	8g	34g
Hazelnuts	16g	6g
Macadamias	8g	14g
Millet	3g	23g
Peanuts	27g	60g
Pecans	10g	56g
Pine nuts/pignolias	16g	12g
Pistachios	24g	11g
Pumpkin Seeds	34g	17g
Rye (one slice of bread)	10g	15g

Protein & Carbohydrate in Nuts & Seeds with no added salt .(per 100g). Continued.

	Protein	Carbohydrate
Sesame seeds	22g	1g
Spelt	6g	60g
Sunflower Seeds	23g	18g
Walnuts	18g	40g

Protein & Sugar in Fruits (100 grams)

	Protein	Sugar
Apple	0.4g	12g
Apricot	1g	8g
Avocado	2g	7g
Blueberries	1g	12g
Blackberries	2g	8g
Blackcurrants	1.5g	9g
Banana	1.2g	20g
Cranberries	0.3g	4g
Cherry	1.4g	13g
Date	3.6g	70g
Fig	1g	18g
Grapefruit (red)	0.9g	7g
Grapes	2.6g	15g
Guava	1g	16g
Gooseberry	1g	9g
Kiwi	1.1g	8g
Kumquat	1g	16g

Protein & Sugar in Fruits (100 grams) Continued

How to Plan Your Meals

	Protein	Sugar
Lemon (with skin)	0.4g	3g
Lime	0.4g	7g
Lychee	1g	17g
Mandarin	0.9g	10g
Mango	1.5g	15g
Melon (red one)	1g	8g
Melon (cantaloupe)	0.9g	6g
Mulberries	1.5g	7g
Nectarine	1.5g	10g
Orange	1g	10g
Papaya	0.8g	8g
Passion Fruit	2.6g	6g
Peach	1g	8g
Pear	0.4g	8g
Persimmon	0.5g	6g
Pineapple	0.4g	12g
Pomegranate	2g	17g
Plum	1.1g	9g
Strawberries	0.8g	5g

Protein on animal products

Fish

In overall, most of the fish fillets or steaks (cooked) contain around 22 grams of protein per 100 grams. Approximately 1.oz per 4.oz (¼lb) of fish.

Eggs

A single poached egg contains 7.5g grams of protein.

Approximately ½.oz per 2 Eggs.

Chicken

Chicken meat cooked contains 30 grams of protein per 100 grams. Approximately 1¼.oz per ¼lb

How to Plan Your Meals

Other Sources of Antioxidant Food

Grapes

The skin and seeds from the grapes all contain polyphenols. This antioxidizing power is ten times greater than vitamin C and E and much easier for the body to absorb.

Olives

The antioxidant property content in Olive fruit and leaf stimulates collagen production which allows the skin to (strengthen) and reduce wrinkles .

Ginkgo

Ginkgo contain flavonols, which are part of the polyphenol family. It improves memory and enhances circulation to the brain, heart, limbs and eyes.

Ginseng

Ginseng has been used for more that 2000 years in China and so it is considered one of the most trusted plants in medical history. Among its properties, ginseng improves health at the cellular level, helps enhance the immune system's resistance to disease and it helps detoxify the body of poisons and waste materials.

Green Tea

Green tea protects the skin's immune system and slows down cellular ageing. It also prevents cancer and protects arteries from clogging.

White Tea

White tea retains more polyphenol that green tea. This is because of the shorter processing time during its oxidation process and therefore provides more anti-oxidation power.

Pomegranate

Its polyphenol antioxidant power is 3 times greater than that of polyphenols from green tea and red wine.

Red Wine

The antioxidant properties of the polyphenol can maintain firmness on the skin.

Royal Jelly

It contains vitamins A,C,D and E, enzymes and antibacterial components. It also contains all of the B complex. Thus helping the immune system to work more efficiently.

Wheat Sprout

It contains a great variety of vitamins, minerals and trace elements. Among those it contains Vitamin A, calcium, phosphorous, potassium, thiamin, riboflavin, niacin and iron.

Sea Vegetables

Have a high antioxidant level that helps protect from radiation and is beneficial to the sensory nerves. They contain a great number of vitamins such as Vitamin A, the B vitamins, vitamin C and vitamin E. They also contain minerals. Among those, bromine, calcium, copper, potassium, selenium, sodium, Zinc and sulphur.

Wheat Grass

Rich nutritional food that contains a great variety of vitamins, minerals and trace elements.

Spirulina

Aids in the protection of the immune system, cholesterol reduction and mineral absorption. It has one of the highest sources of vitamin B 12. It also contains gamma linolenic acid (GLA).

Barley Grass

Contains large amounts of enzymes, beta carotene, magnesium and potassium. It is high in calcium, iron, vitamin B12, vitamin C and flavonoids.

Acerola Berry

Contains the most powerful source of natural vitamin C and bioflavanoids. Among many of it's properties, it allows for a proper colon function.

Index

Alphabetical Index

Index

Index

The Dorian Gray Diet